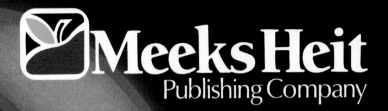

Totally Awesome® Health

Linda Meeks
The Ohio State University

Philip Heit
The Ohio State University

Meeks Heit Publishing Company
Editorial, Sales, and Customer Service
6833 Clark State Road
Blacklick, OH 43004
(614) 939-1111

Director of Editorial: Julie DeVillers
Managing Editor: Ginger Panico
Project Editors: Heather L. Allen, Teri A. Curtis
Director of Illustration: Deborah Rubenstein
Director of Graphics: Elizabeth S. Kim
Graphics Associate: DanniElena Wolfe Hernández
Art Consultant: Jim Brower
Director of Production: Sally Meckling
Designer: Mary Geer
Photographers: Roman Sapecki, Lew Lause
Illustrators: Jennifer King, Dave Odell

Unit 10 outlines emergency care procedures that reflect the standard of knowledge and accepted practices in the United States at the time this book was published. It is the teacher's responsibility to stay informed of changes in emergency care procedures in order to teach current accepted practices. The teacher also can recommend that students gain complete, comprehensive training from courses offered by the American Red Cross.

Printed in the United States of America

   3 4 5 6 7 8 9 10   99

Library of Congress Catalog Number: 98-066101

ISBN: 1-886693-71-4

About Meeks Heit Publishing Company

Professor Linda Meeks   **Dr. Philip Heit**

Linda Meeks and Philip Heit are emeritus professors of Health Education in the College of Education at The Ohio State University. Linda and Philip are America's most widely published health education co-authors. They have collaborated for more than 20 years, co-authoring more than 200 health books that are used by millions of students preschool through college. Together, they have helped state departments of education as well as thousands of school districts develop comprehensive school health education curricula. Their books and curricula are used throughout the United States as well as in Canada, Japan, Mexico, England, Puerto Rico, Spain, Egypt, Jordan, Saudi Arabia, Bermuda, and the Virgin Islands. Linda and Philip train professors as well as educators in state departments of education and school districts. Their book, *Comprehensive School Health Education: Totally Awesome® Strategies for Teaching Health,* is the most widely used book for teacher training in colleges, universities, and school districts. Thousands of teachers throughout the world have participated in their Totally Awesome® Teacher Training Workshops. Linda and Philip have been the keynote speakers for many teacher institutes and wellness conferences. They are personally and professionally committed to the health and well-being of youth.

Contributing Consultant

Susan Wooley, Ph.D., CHES
Executive Director
American School Health Association
Kent, Ohio

Advisory Board

Catherine M. Balsley, Ed.D., CHES
Curriculum Coordinator for
  Comprehensive Health Education
School District of Philadelphia
Philadelphia, Pennsylvania

Gary English, Ph.D., CHES
Associate Professor of Health Education
Department of Health Promotion and
  Human Movement
Ithaca College
Ithaca, New York

Deborah Fortune, Ph.D., CHES
Director of HIV/AIDS Project
Association for the Advancement of
  Health Education
Reston, Virginia

Alison Gardner, M.S., R.D.
Public Health Nutrition Chief
Vermont Department of Health
Burlington, Vermont

Sheryl Gotts, M.S.
Curriculum Specialist
Office of Health and Physical Education
Milwaukee Public Schools
Milwaukee, Wisconsin

David Lohrmann, Ph.D., CHES
Project Director
The Evaluation Consultation Center
Academy for Educational Development
Washington, D.C.

Judy Loper, Ph.D., R.D., L.D.
Director
Central Ohio Nutrition Center
Columbus, Ohio

Deborah Miller, Ph.D., CHES
Professor and Health Coordinator
College/University of Charleston
Charleston, South Carolina

Joanne Owens-Nauslar, Ed.D.
Director of Professional Development
American School Health Association
Kent, Ohio

Linda Peveler, M.S.
Health Teacher
Columbiana Middle School
Shelby County Public Schools
Birmingham, Alabama

LaNaya Ritson, M.S., CHES
Instructor, Department of Health Education
Western Oregon University
Monmouth, Oregon

John Rohwer, Ed.D.
Professor, Department of Health Education
Bethel College
St. Paul, Minnesota

Michael Schaffer, M.A.
Supervisor of Health
  Education K–12
Prince George's County
  Public Schools
Upper Marlboro, Maryland

Sherman Sowby, Ph.D., CHES
Professor, Health Science
California State University at Fresno
Fresno, California

Mae Waters, Ph.D., CHES
Executive Director Comprehensive School
  Health Programs Training Center
Florida State University
Tallahassee, Florida

Dee Wengert, Ph.D., CHES
Professor, Department of Health Science
Towson State University
Towson, Maryland

Medical Reviewers

Donna Bacchi, M.D., M.P.H.
Associate Professor of
  Pediatrics
Director, Division of
  Community Pediatrics
Texas Tech University
  Health Sciences Center
Lubbock, Texas

Albert J. Hart, Jr., M.D.
Mid-Ohio OB-GYN, Inc.
Westerville, Ohio

Reviewers

Kymm Ballard, M.A.
Physical Education, Athletics,
  and Sports Medicine
  Consultant
North Carolina Department
  of Public Instruction
Raleigh, North Carolina

Kay Bridges
Health Educator
Gaston County Public Schools
Gastonia, North Carolina

Reba Bullock, M.Ed.
Health Education Curriculum
  Specialist
Baltimore City Public Schools
Baltimore, Maryland

Anthony S. Catalano, Ph.D.
K–12 Health Coordinator
Melrose Public Schools
Melrose, Massachusetts

Galen Cole, M.P.H., Ph.D.
Division of Health
  Communication
Office of the Director
Centers for Disease Control
  and Prevention
Atlanta, Georgia

Brian Colwell, Ph.D.
Professor
Department of HLKN
Texas A&M University
College Station, Texas

Tommy Fleming, Ph.D.
Director of Health and
  Physical Education
Texas Education Agency
Austin, Texas

Denyce Ford, M.Ed., Ph.D.
Coordinator, Comprehensive
  School Health Education
District of Columbia Public
  Schools
Washington, D.C.

Elizabeth Gallun, M.A.
Supervisor of Drug Programs
Prince George's County
  Public Schools
Upper Marlboro, Maryland

Linda Harrill-Rudisill, M.A.
Chairperson of Health
  Education
Southwest Middle Schools
Gastonia, North Carolina

Janet Henke
Middle School Team Leader
Baltimore County Public
  Schools
Baltimore, Maryland

Russell Henke
Coordinator of Health
Montgomery County Public
  Schools
Rockville, Maryland

Larry Herrold, M.S.
Supervisor, Office of Health
  and Physical Education
  K–12
Baltimore County Schools
Baltimore, Maryland

Susan Jackson, B.S., M.A.
Health Promotion Specialist
Healthworks, Wake Medical
  Center
Raleigh, North Carolina

Joe Leake, CHES
Curriculum Specialist
Baltimore City Public Schools
Baltimore, Maryland

Debra Ogden, M.A.
Coordinator of Health,
  Physical Education, Driver
  Education, and Safe and
  Drug-Free Programs
Collier County Public
  Schools
Naples, Florida

Diane S. Scalise, R.N., M.S.
Coordinator, Health
  Education Services
The School Board of
  Broward County
Fort Lauderdale, Florida

Merita Thompson, Ed.D.
Professor of Health
  Education
Eastern Kentucky University
Richmond, Kentucky

Linda Wright, M.A.
Project Director
HIV/AIDS Education
  Program
District of Columbia
  Public Schools
Washington, D.C.

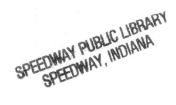

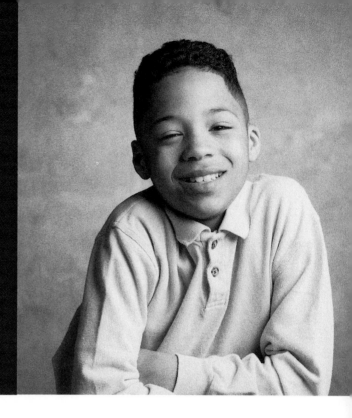

Unit 1

Mental and Emotional Health

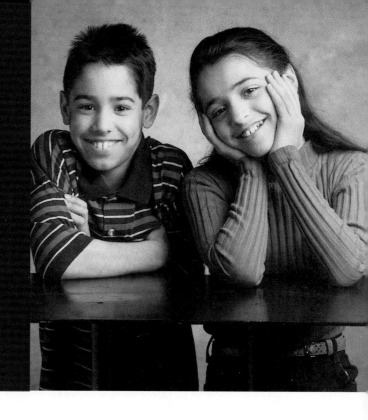

Unit 2

Family and Social Health

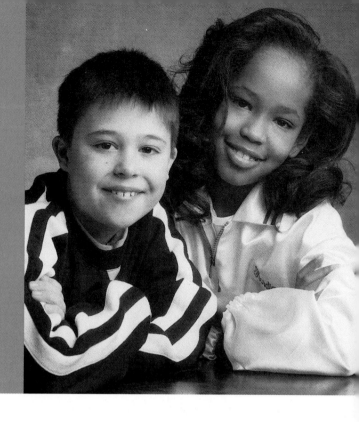

Unit 3

Growth and Development

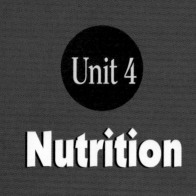

Unit 4
Nutrition

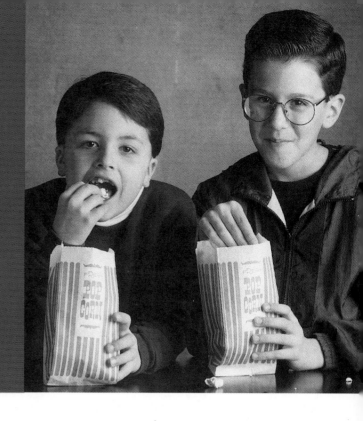

Unit 5

Personal Health and Physical Activity

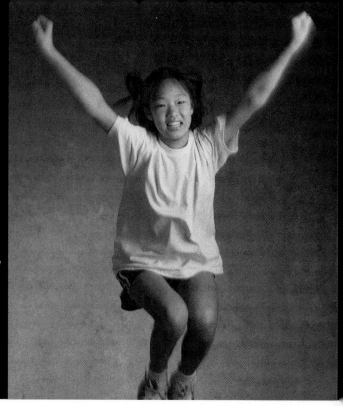

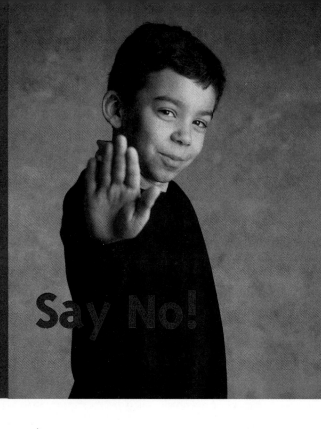

Unit 6

Alcohol, Tobacco, and Other Drugs

Say No!

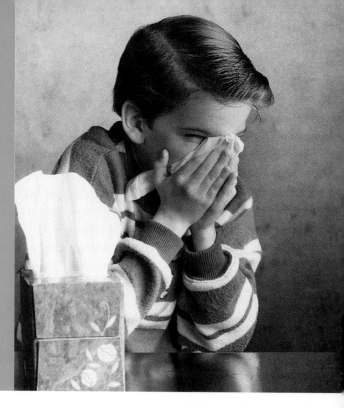

Unit 7

Communicable and Chronic Diseases

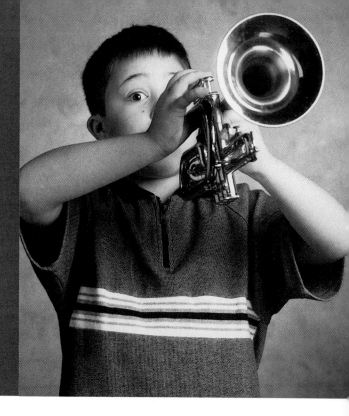

Unit 8

Consumer and Community Health

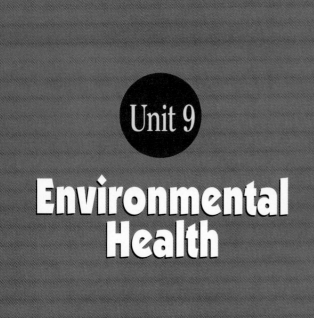

Unit 9

Environmental Health

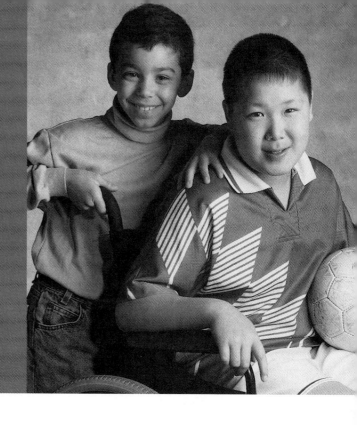

Unit 10

Injury Prevention and Safety

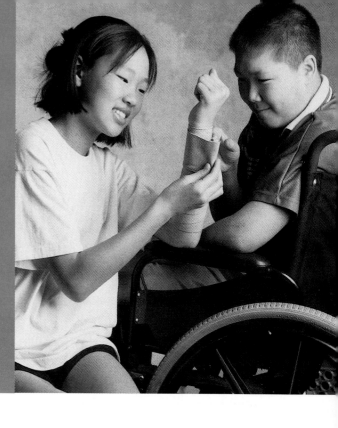

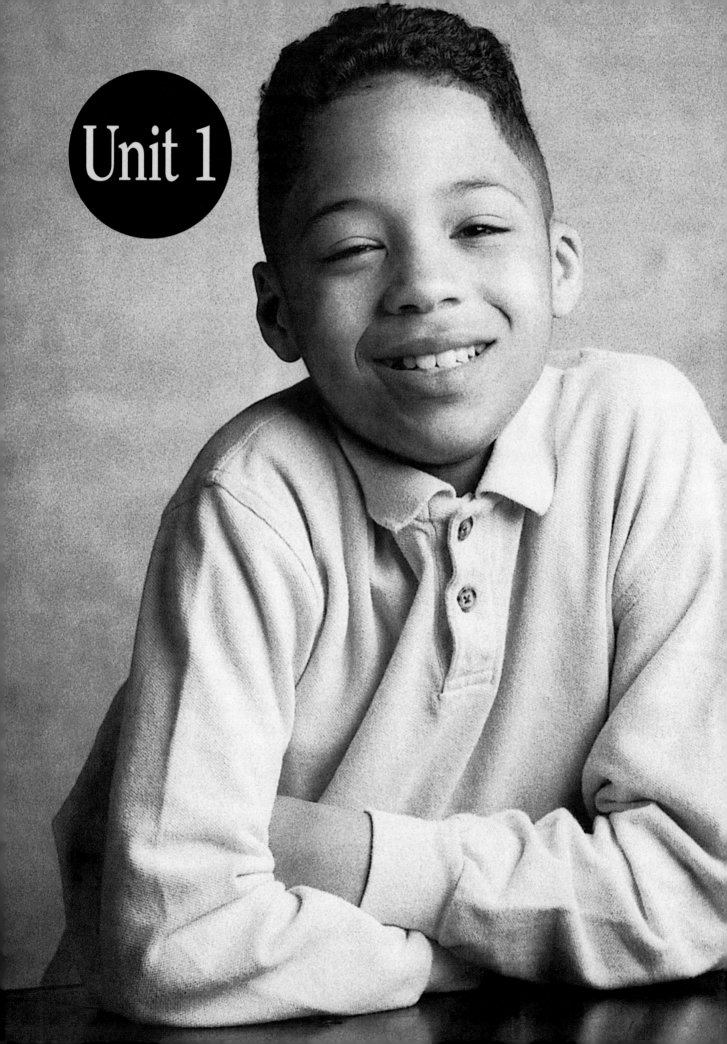

Unit 1

Mental and Emotional Health

Get "High on Health"

Vocabulary

health: the state of your body and mind and the way you get along with others.

wellness: the highest level of health you can reach.

healthful behavior: an action that increases the level of health for you and others.

risk behavior: an action that can be harmful to you and others.

health knowledge: an awareness of facts about health.

life skill: a healthful action you learn and practice for the rest of your life.

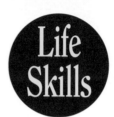

Life Skills

- I will take responsibility for my health.
- I will practice life skills for health.

You can get "high on health." When you get "high on health," you enjoy life to its fullest. You are at your best and reach your potential. To get "high on health," you need to have up-to-date health information. You need to use your health knowledge to choose actions that promote health for you and others. This textbook provides up-to-date health information. It describes ways to put your knowledge into action so that you can get "high on health."

The Lesson Objectives

- Explain how you can achieve high-level wellness.
- Explain why you need to have health knowledge.
- List the Ten Areas of Health.
- Explain how to take responsibility for your health.
- Explain when and how to use a health behavior contract.

How Can I Achieve High-Level Wellness?

Health is the state of your body and mind and the way you get along with others. There are three kinds of health. Physical health is the state of your body. You can improve physical health by getting plenty of exercise, rest, and sleep. Mental health is the state of your mind and the way you express feelings. You can improve mental health by keeping your mind sharp. Read often and work to solve problems. You can also improve mental health by learning how to express feelings in healthful ways. Social health is the state of your relationships with others. You can improve social health by using table manners and treating others with respect.

Wellness is the highest level of health you can reach. Look at *The Wellness Scale.* One end of *The Wellness Scale* stands for high-level wellness. You can reach high-level wellness by: 1) practicing healthful behaviors; 2) avoiding risk behaviors; 3) avoiding risk situations.

A **healthful behavior** is an action that increases the level of health for you and others. Examples are eating a healthful breakfast and getting plenty of exercise.

The other end of *The Wellness Scale* stands for injury, illness, and premature death. *Premature death* is a death that happens before the usual time. Practicing risk behaviors can cause injury, illness, and premature death. A **risk behavior** is an action that can be harmful to you and others. Examples are riding double on a bike and drinking alcohol. Risk situations also can cause injury, illness, and premature death. A *risk situation* is a condition that can harm your health. An example is riding in a car with a driver who is speeding.

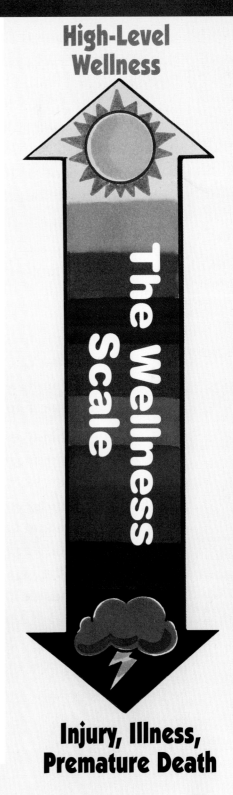

High-Level Wellness

The Wellness Scale

Injury, Illness, Premature Death

Why Do I Need to Have Health Knowledge?

Health knowledge is an awareness of facts about health. You need health knowledge to tell the difference between healthful behaviors and risk behaviors. You need health knowledge to know about risk situations you must avoid. This textbook is arranged into ten units. Each unit contains health knowledge about one area of health. Read the chart on the next page and learn about the Ten Areas of Health.

A single healthful behavior, a risk behavior, and a risk situation can each affect any one or more areas of health. For example, running is a healthful behavior. Running improves the condition of your heart and lungs and helps make your bones strong (Growth and Development). Running helps you relax (Mental and Emotional Health). Running can be enjoyed with a family member or friend (Family and Social Health). Running, a healthful behavior, improves many areas of health.

Cigarette smoking is a risk behavior. Chemicals in cigarette smoke damage lung cells and raise heart rate (Growth and Development). Smoking makes the chances of heart disease and cancer greater (Communicable and Chronic Diseases). Cigarette smoke bothers other people (Family and Social Health). Smoking cigarettes, a risk behavior, harms many areas of health.

Whole Person Health

Health experts have studied whole person health. They know that any one behavior can affect you as a whole person. Suppose you change one risk behavior to a healthful behavior. For example, maybe you never eat breakfast with cereal, orange juice, and milk. This is a risk behavior. Then you change this to a healthful behavior. You have breakfast with cereal, orange juice, and milk. You have more energy for school and play. The cereal helps you have a daily bowel movement. The orange juice gives you vitamins to help against disease. The milk has minerals for bones. You changed one risk behavior and you got several benefits.

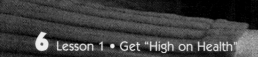

Ten Areas of Health

Mental and Emotional Health

includes how you make decisions, how you express feelings, ways you keep your mind sharp, ways you deal with stress.

Family and Social Health

includes how you relate with your family, ways you make decisions with friends, how you handle conflict.

Growth and Development

includes ways to care for your body systems, actions that help you age in a healthful way, how you learn best.

Nutrition

includes food choices to have a healthy body, to prevent disease, and to have a healthful weight.

Personal Health and Physical Activity

includes why you need checkups, how to be well-groomed, why you need plenty of exercise, how to make a fitness plan, how to be a good sport.

Alcohol, Tobacco, and Other Drugs

includes how to use medicine in safe ways; why you should stay away from alcohol, tobacco, and illegal drugs; how to resist pressure to use drugs.

Communicable and Chronic Diseases

includes habits that help prevent diseases, symptoms and treatment for diseases, what to know about HIV.

Consumer and Community Health

includes how to check out sources of health information; how to choose safe and healthful products; how to make choices about time, money, and entertainment; descriptions of community health helpers; what to know about health careers.

Environmental Health

includes how to keep the air, land, and water clean and safe; how to stay away from noise; how to conserve energy and resources.

Injury Prevention and Safety

includes safety rules for different situations, ways to protect yourself in awful weather, ways to protect yourself from violence, first aid skills.

How Do I Take Responsibility for My Health?

As you read this book, you will receive health knowledge for each of the ten health areas. But having health knowledge is not enough. You take responsibility for health by practicing life skills. A **life skill** is a healthful action you learn and practice for the rest of your life. Here is a list of life skills for each of the ten health areas. Each life skill begins with "I will" because you must be "willing" to practice life skills.

Mental and Emotional Health

- I will take responsibility for my health.
- I will practice life skills for health.
- I will make responsible decisions.
- I will use resistance skills when necessary.
- I will show good character.
- I will communicate in healthful ways.
- I will choose behaviors to have a healthy mind.
- I will have a plan for stress.
- I will bounce back from hard times.

Family and Social Health

- I will show respect for all people.
- I will encourage other people to take responsibility for their health.
- I will settle conflict in healthful ways.
- I will work to have healthful friendships.
- I will work to have healthful family relationships.
- I will adjust to family changes in healthful ways.
- I will prepare for future relationships.
- I will practice abstinence.

Growth and Development

- I will care for my body systems.
- I will learn the stages of the life cycle.
- I will accept how my body changes as I grow.
- I will choose habits for healthful growth and aging.
- I will be glad that I am unique.
- I will discover my learning style.

Nutrition

- I will eat the correct number of servings from the Food Guide Pyramid.
- I will follow the Dietary Guidelines.
- I will read food labels.
- I will eat healthful meals and snacks.
- I will choose healthful foods if I eat at fast food restaurants.
- I will protect myself and others from germs in foods and beverages.
- I will use table manners.
- I will stay at a healthful weight.
- I will work on skills to prevent eating disorders.

Personal Health and Physical Activity

- I will have regular checkups.
- I will help my parents or guardian keep my personal health record.
- I will follow a dental health plan.
- I will be well-groomed.
- I will get plenty of physical activity.
- I will follow safety rules for sports and games.
- I will prevent injuries during physical activity.
- I will get enough rest and sleep.

Alcohol, Tobacco, and Other Drugs

- I will use over-the-counter (OTC) and prescription drugs in safe ways.
- I will tell ways to get help for someone who uses drugs in harmful ways.
- I will say NO if someone offers me a harmful drug.
- I will not drink alcohol.
- I will not use tobacco.
- I will protect myself from secondhand smoke.
- I will not be involved in illegal drug use.

Communicable and Chronic Diseases

- I will choose habits that prevent the spread of germs.
- I will recognize symptoms and get treatment for communicable diseases.
- I will choose habits that prevent heart disease.
- I will choose habits that prevent cancer.
- I will tell ways to care for asthma and allergies.
- I will tell ways to care for chronic (lasting) health conditions.
- I will learn facts about HIV and AIDS.

Consumer and Community Health

- I will check out sources of health information.
- I will check ways technology, media, and culture influence health choices.
- I will choose safe and healthful products.
- I will spend time and money wisely.
- I will choose healthful entertainment.
- I will cooperate with community and school health helpers.
- I will learn about health careers.

Environmental Health

- I will help protect my environment.
- I will keep the air, water, and land clean and safe.
- I will keep noise at a safe level.
- I will not waste energy and resources.
- I will help keep my environment friendly.

Injury Prevention and Safety

- I will follow safety rules for my home and school.
- I will follow safety rules for biking, walking, and swimming.
- I will follow safety rules for riding in a car.
- I will follow safety rules for weather conditions.
- I will protect myself from people who might harm me.
- I will follow safety rules to protect myself from violence.
- I will stay away from gangs.
- I will not carry a weapon.
- I will be skilled in first aid.

How Can I Use a Health Behavior Contract?

A *health behavior contract* is a written plan to practice a life skill. Use a health behavior contract to start the new habit of practicing a life skill. There are four steps to follow to make a health behavior contract.

Health Behavior Contract

Name: _____ **Date:** _____

Life Skill: I will get plenty of physical activity.

Effect On My Health: Physical activity helps make my heart muscle and my bones strong. I can keep a healthful weight if I get plenty of physical activity. I can keep from being stressed.

My Plan: I will take part in physical activity for at least thirty minutes each day. I will take part in high-energy physical activity to keep my heart strong. I will write the physical activities in which I will take part next week on my calendar. I will place a star by the days of the week that I stick to my plan.

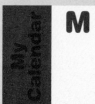

My Calendar	M	T	W	Th	F	S	S

How My Plan Worked: I will talk about how my plan worked. For example, if I skip a day of physical activity, I will tell why.

Four Steps to Follow to Make a Health Behavior Contract

1. Tell the life skill you want to practice.

2. Tell how the life skill will affect your health.

3. Describe a plan you will follow and how you will keep track of your progress.

4. Tell how your plan worked.

Stay "High on Health"

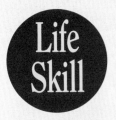

Life Skill I will practice life skills for health.

Materials: A balloon

Directions: Read through the list of life skills on pages 8–9. Try to remember as many life skills as you can.

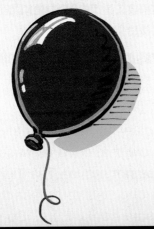

Activity

1. Stand with your classmates in a clear area of your classroom.
2. One classmate names a life skill and taps the balloon high in the air toward a second classmate.
3. The second classmate names a different life skill and taps the balloon high in the air toward a third classmate. Continue as long as possible. Classmates stay "high on health" by naming a life skill and tapping the balloon before it drops.

Lesson 1

Review

Vocabulary

Write a separate sentence using each of the vocabulary words listed on page 4.

Health Content

Write answers to the following:

1. What are the three kinds of health? **page 5**
2. How can you reach high-level wellness? **page 5**
3. Why do you need to have health knowledge? **page 6**
4. How can you take responsibility for your health? **page 8**
5. How can you use a health behavior contract? **page 10**

Stick to Responsible Decisions

Vocabulary

responsible decision: a decision that is safe, healthful, and follows laws and family guidelines.

respect: thinking highly of someone.

good character: telling the truth, showing respect, and being fair.

peer pressure: the influence that peers try to have on your decisions.

wrong decision: a decision that is harmful, unsafe, and that breaks laws or family guidelines.

resistance skills: skills that help you resist pressure to make a wrong decision.

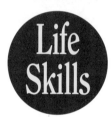 Life Skills

- **I will make responsible decisions.**
- **I will use resistance skills when necessary.**

Have you used "super glue" to make something stick? If you have, you know that once you use "super glue" on something, it does not move. The ingredients in "super glue" are very strong. As you reach the teen years, you might get pressure from others. Someone you know might try to pull you away from doing what is right. You will need to be strong like "super glue." You will need to stick to responsible decisions.

The Lesson Objectives

- Explain how to make responsible decisions.
- List six questions to ask before you make a decision.
- List seven resistance skills you can use to resist pressure to make a wrong decision.
- Explain why a peer might pressure you to make a wrong decision.

How Can I Make Responsible Decisions?

A decision is a choice you make. To achieve high-level wellness, you must make responsible decisions. A **responsible decision** is a decision that is safe, healthful, and follows laws and family guidelines. When you make responsible decisions, you show respect for yourself and others. **Respect** is thinking highly of someone. You show good character when you make responsible decisions. **Good character** is telling the truth, showing respect, and being fair.

Guidelines for Making Responsible Decisions™ are questions you ask to help you make a responsible decision.

Suppose you have to make a decision. Fill in each blank with what you might do. Then answer each of the six questions. Your answers to all six questions should be YES. Then you know your decision is responsible. Suppose you answer NO to one or more questions. Then you know your decision is not responsible.

1. Is is healthful to _____?
2. Is it safe to _____?
3. Do I follow rules and laws if I _____?
4. Do I show respect for myself and others if I _____?
5. Do I follow my family's guidelines if I _____?
6. Do I show good character if I _____?

Ask a Trusted Adult for Suggestions

Your parents, guardian, or other trusted adults can guide you. Ask for suggestions when you have a hard decision. They can help you explore some of your choices. They might think of possible decisions you have not thought of. They can discuss the results of decisions with you. There might be facts or results about which you do not know.

Guidelines for Making Responsible Decisions™

How Can I Use Resistance Skills?

A *peer* is a person who is about your age. **Peer pressure** is the influence that peers try to have on your decisions. Peers might influence you to make responsible decisions. For example, your peers might want you to eat breakfast and study for tests. Some peers might try to get you to make wrong decisions. A **wrong decision** is a decision that is harmful, unsafe, and that breaks laws or family guidelines. For example, peers might ask that you join them and hitchhike. Hitchhiking is not safe. Hitchhiking is illegal. Your parents or guardian do not want you to hitchhike. Peers who want you to hitchhike are trying to get you to make a wrong decision.

Resistance skills are skills that help you resist pressure to make a wrong decision. Try to remember the resistance skills that are listed in the margin. Use resistance skills if peers pressure you to make a wrong decision.

Suppose a peer does not know or understand the possible outcomes of a decision. The peer might not realize that a decision might result in actions that are harmful, unsafe, or break laws or family guidelines. If you explain the possible results, the peer should back off. But suppose the peer does not back off. This peer might pressure you to make a wrong decision so you will get into trouble. This peer might pressure you to make a wrong decision because he or she makes wrong decisions. You can be certain of one thing. This peer does not respect you or care about you. A peer who respects you and cares about you does not pressure you to make wrong decisions.

Resistance Skills

1. Say NO in a firm voice.
2. Give reasons for saying NO.
3. Be certain your behavior matches your words.
4. Avoid situations in which there will be pressure to make wrong decisions.
5. Avoid being with people who make wrong decisions.
6. Tell an adult right away if you are pressured to make a decision that results in actions that break laws.
7. Encourage others to make responsible decisions.

"Catch" a Peer Being Responsible

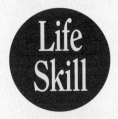

Life Skill

I will make responsible decisions.

Materials: Camera (optional), paper, markers

Directions: Complete this activity to learn ways you and your peers can use positive peer pressure to help each other.

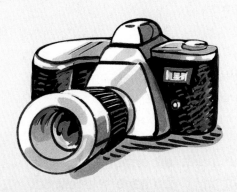

Activity

1. **"Catch" a peer trying to influence you or other peers in a positive way.** For example, you might "catch" a peer who says, "Let's sit in the nonsmoking section of the restaurant." You might "catch" a peer who says, "Let's ride bikes after school today."

2. **(Optional) Take a snapshot of the peer who has responsible behavior.**

3. **Make an award to recognize this peer for the positive influence he or she has on you and others.** Use the paper and markers. Create a name for the award. Design the award with a place for your peer's name.

4. **Share the award with your classmates.**

Lesson 2

Review

Vocabulary

Write a separate sentence using each of the vocabulary words listed on page 12.

Health Content

Write answers to the following:

1. How can you make responsible decisions? **page 13**
2. What are six questions to ask before you make a decision? **page 13**
3. When is a decision a wrong one? **page 14**
4. What are seven resistance skills you can use to resist pressure to make a wrong decision? **page 14**
5. Why might a peer pressure you to make a wrong decision? **page 14**

Keep Good Character with You

Vocabulary

personality: a blend of the different traits you have.

self-respect: the good feelings you have about yourself when you behave in responsible ways.

self-control: the degree to which you regulate your behavior.

good character: telling the truth, showing respect, and being fair.

responsible value: a belief that guides you to behave in responsible ways.

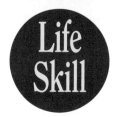

Life Skill

● **I will show good character.**

Your **personality** is a blend of the different traits you have. Suppose someone you know described your personality. This person might talk about your physical traits. He or she might talk about your mental and emotional traits. He or she might talk about your social traits. And he or she might say if you have self-respect and good character.

The Lesson Objectives

● List traits that are part of a person's personality.

● List and discuss ways to develop self-respect.

● List and discuss ways to show you have good character.

How Do I Develop Self-Respect?

Self-respect is the good feelings you have about yourself when you behave in responsible ways. Self-respect is an important part of mental health. These tips help you develop and keep your self-respect.

1. **Do what is expected of you.** There are jobs that you are expected to complete. Complete these jobs even when you do not feel like it. Later, you will feel good about yourself because you have done what was expected of you.

2. **Choose responsible behavior.** Good feelings about yourself come from knowing that your actions were good or responsible.

3. **Use self-control.** Self-control is the degree to which you regulate your behavior. It is your willingness to stick to something difficult. Suppose a test is difficult for you. Your classmate's paper is in view and you could sneak a peek at her answers. Self-control is needed to keep your eyes on your own paper. You rely on yourself for the correct answer. Then the score you get on the test is fair. If you do well, you can feel good about the score. If you do not do well, you study harder the next time. The extra effort you make helps you have good feelings. You are responsible.

4. **Work hard.** Always try as hard as you can. Do not give up easily when something is difficult for you. Laziness or taking shortcuts will not help you develop self-respect. You have good feelings about yourself when you do not give up and you finally finish what you wanted to do.

5. **Correct wrong actions.** No one is perfect all the time. Suppose you make a mistake and do something wrong. Do not overlook your wrong actions. Do not try to cover up what you have done or hope you can get away with it. Take responsibility for your actions. Apologize and feel real sorrow. Do whatever you can to correct wrong actions. Promise yourself and others that you will not do the same wrong action again on purpose. This is the only way to keep your self-respect. It is the only way to keep the respect of others. Other people can forgive you when you own up to wrong actions. They know that no one is perfect.

How Can I Show I Have Good Character?

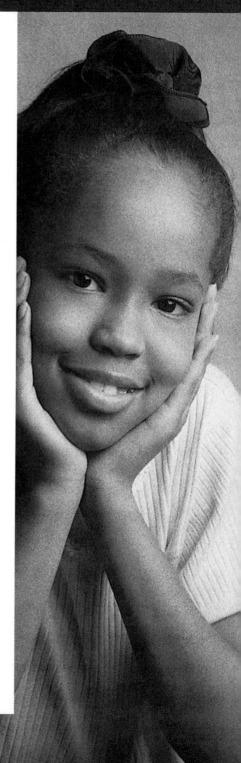

Good character is telling the truth, showing respect, and being fair. A person with good character acts on responsible values. A **responsible value** is a belief that guides you to behave in responsible ways. You show others you have good character when you resist temptation. Let's look at some ways to show you have good character.

Tell the truth. You show others you have good character when you tell the truth. You cannot have good character and tell lies—even little ones. Suppose a friend asks you to come over after school. You are not supposed to go to a friend's house if a parent or guardian will not be there. You could lie to your parents or guardian and say your friend's parent or guardian will be there. Or you could hope your parent or guardian does not ask.

But neither of these actions show good character. Neither action is honest. You must tell the truth even when it is hard. Remember this fact, too. You must encourage other people to tell the truth. You have bad character if you ask other people to lie.

Be fair. You show others you have good character when you are fair. Remember The Golden Rule. Treat others as you expect to be treated. Suppose you buy something at a store and the clerk gives you too much change back. Should you keep the extra change? Of course not. You must tell the clerk and pay the correct amount. This action is fair. This is how you would expect to be treated.

Show respect for others. You show others you have good character when you show respect for them. You do not walk over friends as if they were a doormat. You do not put them down or belittle them. You listen to what they have to say. You do not have to have your own way all the time. When you are with friends, you show others respect. You do not tell cruel jokes about people who are different. You do not make snide remarks about other people.

Suppose someone you know tells a joke about someone who is different. It might be someone of a different race or culture than you are. You know the joke is not funny. You do not laugh at the joke. You do not go along with actions that show disrespect for others.

Complete your share of the workload. You show others you have good character when you complete your share of the workload. For example, you might be assigned a group project at school. Each person in your group is expected to contribute to the project. One person in your group is willing to do most of the work. You could slide and do very little. But trying to get out of your share of the work is a way of cheating. When you have good character, you are willing to be a team player. You pitch in and help when work must be done. You do work with a cheerful attitude. You thank others for doing their share of the workload.

Show you are grateful. You show others you have good character when you are grateful. *Gratitude* is a feeling of thanks for a favor or for something that makes you happy. Take notice of the many things for which you can be thankful. Express your gratitude to others. Do not overlook your parents or guardian. They need to be thanked for their efforts. Do not complain. When something is not as you want it, take actions to change it. Work to gain an understanding of things you do not like that cannot be changed.

Choose Role Models Who Show Good Character

A *role model* is a person whose behavior other people copy. Think about the people you might copy. Have you ever wanted to be like a professional athlete? Have you ever wanted to be like an actor? Have you ever worn a shirt with the name of a musical group on it? It is OK to want to pitch like your favorite baseball pitcher. It is OK to enjoy the character played by your favorite actor. It is OK to have a favorite musical group. You admire the skills of these people. But do further checking. It is not OK to copy the behavior of someone who does not have good character.

Character Coat of Armor

Activity

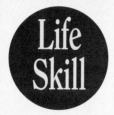

Life Skill

I will show good character.

Materials: Poster board, markers, scissors, heavy string

Directions: Complete the following activity to learn why you need to wear your character coat of armor at all times.

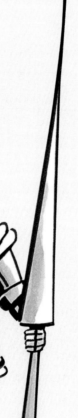

1. **Cut a piece of armor out of poster board.** Attach string to your piece of armor so that it can be worn.

2. **Use markers and write words describing character on the coat of armor.** Write at least ten words. Some words you might write are: honest, fair, hard worker, and responsible.

3. **Think of a situation that might tempt someone your age to do something wrong.** Write this situation on an index card. Give the index card to your teacher. Your teacher will shuffle the index cards.

4. **Put on your character coat of armor.** Your teacher will give you one of the index cards upon which a tempting situation is written. Remember, you are wearing your character coat of armor. Think of ways to deal with this situation that show you have good character.

5. **When it is your turn, share your answer with your class-mates.** Tell why you need good character in tempting situations.

6. **Review the words that your classmates wrote on their coat of armor.** Make a list of all the words on a sheet of paper. Take your list home and review it with your parents or guardian.

Use... Guidelines for Making Responsible Decisions™

Some classmates think it would be cool to smoke a cigar. They dare you to steal three cigars from the store. They say they will talk to the clerk so the clerk will not see you steal the cigars.

Use a separate sheet of paper. Answer "yes" or "no" to each of the following questions. Explain each answer.

1. Is it healthful for you to steal the cigars?
2. Is it safe for you to steal the cigars?
3. Do you follow rules and laws if you steal the cigars?
4. Do you show respect for yourself and others if you steal the cigars?
5. Do you follow your family's guidelines if you steal the cigars?
6. Do you show good character if you steal the cigars?

What is the responsible decision to make?

Lesson 3

Review

Vocabulary

Write a separate sentence using each of the vocabulary words listed on page 16.

Health Content

Write answers to the following:

1. What traits make up a person's personality? **page 16**
2. What are five ways to develop self-respect? **page 17**
3. What should you do if you do something wrong? **page 17**
4. What are five ways to show others you have good character? **pages 18–19**
5. What can you do if something is not the way you want it to be? **page 19**

Put Together the Mind-Body Connection

Vocabulary

communication: an exchange of information with others.

emotions: the feelings you have inside you.

mind-body connection: the idea that your thoughts and feelings have an effect on your body.

I-message: a statement that includes a behavior, the effect of the behavior, and the feeling that results.

mental alertness: the sharpness of your mind.

boredom: the state of being restless because you have no interests.

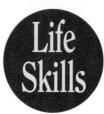

Life Skills

- I will communicate in healthful ways.
- I will choose behaviors to have a healthy mind.

Think of your health as a large puzzle made of many pieces. Some puzzle pieces keep the mind sharp. Some help you communicate and express emotions. Others keep your body strong. If a puzzle piece is missing, you do not get total health. If the puzzle pieces do not fit or work together, you do not get total health.

The Lesson Objectives

- List ten skills you need to communicate with others.
- Explain how to manage your emotions.
- Discuss ways emotions can affect your health.
- Put together I-messages to express feelings.
- Tell ways to keep your mind alert.

What Skills Do I Need to Communicate with Others?

Communication is an exchange of information with others. There are many ways to communicate. One way is writing. Another way is using signals. A third way is talking.

There are two parts of communication. These two parts are giving out information and taking in information. Communication involves expressing yourself clearly to others. Other people are then able to understand what you have said. Communication also involves listening. If you listen well, you know exactly what others are saying to you. You can better understand their feelings.

Some people communicate well. They have learned to say exactly what they mean. They listen carefully. They practice skills that will help them communicate. People who talk and listen well improve their physical, mental, and emotional health.

Communication Checkout

Rate yourself on these skills.

1. I speak loudly enough for others to hear me.
2. I speak clearly and choose words carefully.
3. I am able to express feelings.
4. I act in ways that go together with what I say.
5. I listen carefully when others speak.
6. I watch the actions of a person who speaks to me.
7. I make sure others know that I am listening.
8. I remember what is said.
9. I am careful to repeat correctly what others say.
10. I do not repeat what others trust me to keep secret.

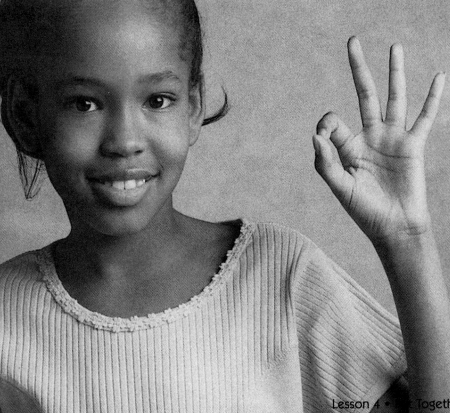

How Can I Manage My Emotions?

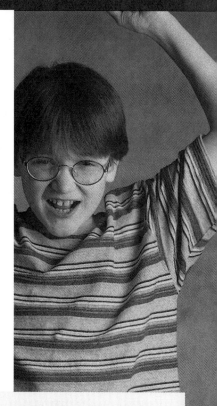

Your **emotions** are the feelings you have inside you. At different times, you have different emotions. You might feel: afraid to give a report in class; angry if a friend gossips about you; proud when you receive a good grade on your health test; sad when your pet is sick or dies.

For good mental health, it is important to know when and how to express your emotions. There are four questions you can answer to help manage your emotions.

1. What is it that I am feeling?
2. Why do I feel this way?
3. What are some ways that I might express how I am feeling?
4. How can I express my feelings in a healthful way?

Test Your Emotion IQ

Suppose you are watching your favorite TV program and leave to get an apple. When you return, your sister has changed the channel. You tell your sister that you were watching your favorite program. She refuses to turn the channel back to the program you were watching.

1. How are you feeling? **Angry**
2. Why are you feeling this way? **Your sister will not turn the channel back to the program.**
3. What are some ways you might express your feelings? **You might raise your voice at your sister and call her unkind names.**

You might feel angry, but choose to keep your angry feelings to yourself.

You might talk with your sister and tell her why you are angry.

4. How can you express your anger in a healthful way?

Calling your sister unkind names will harm your relationship with her.

Keeping your angry feelings to yourself is OK at times. But keeping angry feelings inside for a long time can harm health.

Explaining why you are angry opens up the lines of communication. This action gets the best results.

How Can My Emotions Affect My Health?

There is a mind-body connection about which you should know. The **mind-body connection** is the idea that your thoughts and feelings have an effect on your body. In fact, some health experts say that if you describe what you are thinking and feeling you can predict what can happen inside your body. Some examples will help you better understand the mind-body connection.

Suppose you are feeling rushed. You believe you do not have enough time to get things done. Your mind is racing. How might your thoughts and feelings affect what is happening in your body? Some health experts say that when your mind races and rushes, so does your body. Your heart rate and blood pressure might increase.

Suppose you keep angry feelings bottled up inside you. You do not allow your anger to get out. When it finally does, you explode. Some health experts say that when you let pressure build up in your mind, your body does, too. Your blood pressure increases. You are more at risk for stroke. A stroke occurs when a blood vessel in the brain bursts.

Suppose you are depressed. You feel down most of the time. Some health experts say that when you feel down, your body shuts down, too. The white blood cells that fight disease shut down. Then pathogens in your body multiply. These pathogens can cause disease. You get colds and flu more often. You miss more days of school. You feel tired and lack energy.

Warning: Not Expressing Emotions Can Harm Health

- Pay attention to what you are thinking and feeling.

- Take notice of how your thoughts and feelings affect your body functions.

- Protect your body by expressing your feelings in healthful ways.

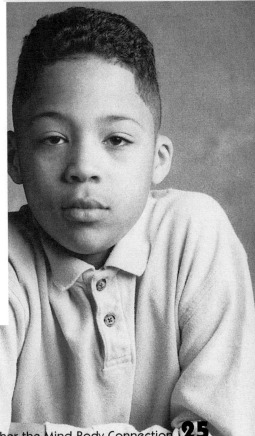

"Wake-Up Call"

Activity

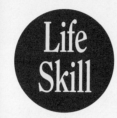

Life Skill

I will communicate in healthful ways.

Materials: Alarm clock, chairs

Directions: Review the information about the mind-body connection. Then follow the steps below to see how the mind-body connection works.

1. **Arrange the classroom as if you were going to play musical chairs.** There will be one less chair to sit on than you have classmates.

2. **The teacher will set the alarm to go off.**

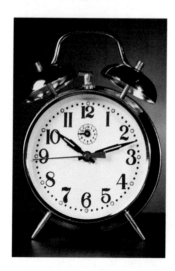

3. **One classmate will name an emotion such as anger.** This classmate will name an emotion that is not being expressed. Or the classmate might name an emotion that is being expressed in a harmful way. For example, expressing anger by fighting.

4. **Then all classmates will walk around the class and wait for the alarm to go off.** The alarm is a "wake-up call." The body responds to the ways you are thinking and feeling. The body sends you a signal or "wake-up call" telling you to take care of yourself. For example, you might have a headache or stomachache. These body symptoms might be a "wake-up call." They might warn you that it is time to deal with certain thoughts and feelings.

5. **When the alarm goes off, classmates will each try to find a chair.**

6. **The classmate who does not find a chair must say one way the body might be out of balance.** For example, the classmate might say, "I feel rushed and have high blood pressure."

How Do I Put Together an I-Message?

One way to share feelings with others is to use an I-message. An **I-message** is a statement that includes a behavior, the effect of the behavior, and the feeling that results. Think about the following example.

You help a friend with his paper route after school. With your help, your friend can finish his paper route early and can get to baseball practice on time. You do not want to help every day but you do not want to tell your friend. Today you tell your friend you will meet him in about fifteen minutes. However, you do not plan to meet your friend. Your friend expects you to do what you said you will do. But you do not. You do not express your feelings in an open and honest way.

Put together an I-message to express your feelings. (Check out the I-message in the margin.) Start with naming the behavior. Then tell how the behavior affects you. Go one step further and tell how this makes you feel.

An I-message is a responsibility message. You take responsibility for what you are feeling. You do not blame someone else. The other person can respond to you. Think about the effect of a blame message. You are selfish to ask me to help you with your paper route every day. The other person will feel as though she is being attacked and might attack back.

An I-message does not make a person put up his or her guard. You do not want people to feel guarded around you. You want people to feel comfortable. When you use I-messages, you have more friends.

Put Together an I-Message

The behavior
When I help with your paper route...

The effect
...I do not have time for things I want to do...

The feelings that result
...and I get angry.

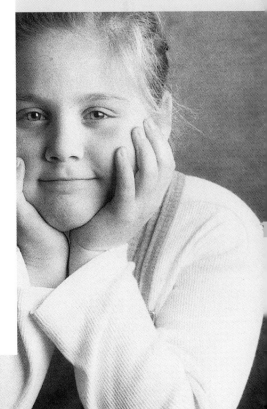

How Can I Keep My Mind Alert?

Mental alertness is the sharpness of your mind. You can keep your mind sharp in two ways. First, you can use your mind often. This is how you keep your mind in good condition. Think about ways you can use your mind. Read books in which you learn new facts. Remember facts and store them in your brain. Then try to think again about these facts at a later time. Work to add new words to your vocabulary. Complete crossword puzzles or play word games.

Remember the mind-body connection. Health experts say that you must keep your body in top form to be mentally alert. Choose a drug-free lifestyle. Do not drink alcohol. Alcohol depresses brain cells. Alcohol also kills brain cells. Drinking alcohol can affect mental alertness.

Do not smoke cigarettes. Carbon monoxide is a poisonous gas in cigarette smoke. If you smoke, carbon monoxide enters your blood. Your circulation will not be as good as it should be. To be mentally alert, you need to have good circulation.

Get plenty of physical activity. Physical activity improves circulation. Your brain will get the oxygen it needs to do its work. Eat a healthful, balanced diet. Do not skip meals, especially breakfast. When you skip breakfast, your blood sugar level drops. Your brain does not have the nutrients it needs to work. You will not think as clearly.

Talk to adults about facts and situations. Adults can ask you questions that make you think. Your mind stays sharp when you think things through. You can share reasons for your answers.

Cures for Boredom

Boredom is the state of being restless because you have no interests. You feel like there is nothing to do. Don't just hang around and do nothing. A cure to boredom is to find a new interest. Get involved in a club or school activity. Try a new sport or hobby. Learn a foreign language. Read a book. Talk to your parents or guardian if you often feel bored.

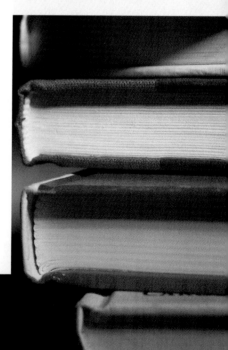

Brain Foods

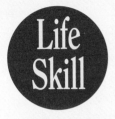

Life Skill

I will choose behaviors to have a healthy mind.

Materials: Magazines with pictures of foods, poster board, scissors, glue

Directions: Read the information about the B vitamins. Then complete the following to plan to eat brain foods for brain power.

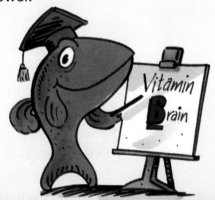

What to Know About B Vitamins

Your brain is part of your nervous system. Vitamin B_1 and vitamin B_{12} keep your nervous system in top condition. Foods rich in the B vitamins include: poultry, fish, eggs, cheese, milk, whole-grain cereal, whole-grain bread, dried beans, and pasta.

1. **Divide the class into groups of five students.**
2. **Each group will cut out pictures of foods rich in vitamin B from magazines.**
3. **Each group will glue their pictures of brain foods to a sheet of poster board.**
4. **Each group will share its poster of brain foods with the class.**
5. **Name other ways to keep the brain in top condition.**

Activity

Lesson 4

Review

Vocabulary

Write a separate sentence using each of the vocabulary words listed on page 22.

Health Content

Write answers to the following:

1. What are ten skills you need to communicate with others? **page 23**
2. What are four questions to answer to help manage your emotions? **page 24**
3. What are ways your emotions can affect your health? **page 25**
4. What are the parts of an I-message? **page 27**
5. How can I keep my mind alert? **page 28**

Reduce That Stress

Vocabulary

stress: the body's reaction to the demands of daily living.

stressor: something that causes stress.

eustress: a healthful response to a stressor.

distress: unsuccessful coping or a harmful response to a stressor.

stress management skills: ways to reduce harmful effects of body changes caused by a stressor.

positive attitude: a positive way of thinking and seeing things.

support network: the group of people who care about you.

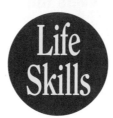

Life Skills

- **I will have a plan for stress.**
- **I will bounce back from hard times.**

You have probably been in some of these situations: you have a big championship game; you give a report in front of class; you have a disagreement with a friend; you have a difficult test coming up. Situations such as these can cause you to feel excited, nervous, sad, worried, or tired. These kinds of emotions are signs of stress. **Stress** is the body's reaction to the demands of daily living. To stay healthy, you must know how to lower stress.

The Lesson Objectives

- Talk about body changes that occur if you get stressed out.
- Tell ways to protect your health if you get stressed out.
- Explain how to bounce back from hard times.

What Body Changes Occur If I Get Stressed Out?

A **stressor** is something that causes stress. When you experience a stressor, your body reacts in many ways. Your glands release sugar into your bloodstream. This helps you have more energy. Your heart beats faster. Your breathing rate increases. More blood flows to your muscles to help you move. Your hands might become moist.

Changes that occur in your body as a reaction to stress can be healthful or harmful. The changes stress will cause depends on how long it lasts. Suppose your class is going to have a difficult test. If you feel ready to take the test, you experience eustress. **Eustress** (YOO·stres) is a healthful response to a stressor. Body changes help you perform well. These body changes are not severe. They do not last longer than they are needed.

If you worry a lot about the test, you experience distress. **Distress** is unsuccessful coping or a harmful response to a stressor. Body changes that happen are severe. They get in the way of how you perform. For example, you might get very tired. You might get headaches and stomachaches, and have allergic reactions.

Suppose you get stressed out often. Body changes caused by stress can cause health conditions and diseases. Cancer, heart disease, asthma, and allergies are more common in people who get stressed out often.

People who have health conditions should not get stressed out either. For example, suppose you have had asthma for awhile. Stress can bring on an asthma attack. Suppose you have allergies. Stress might bring out a skin rash.

Stressors Add Up

stressor + stressor + stressor = disease

The death of a family member and the divorce of parents are two major stressors for young people. These stressors can affect health. But smaller stressors can affect health, too. Health experts say that several smaller stressors can add up and have the same effects as a major stressor.

How Can I Protect My Health If I Get Stressed Out?

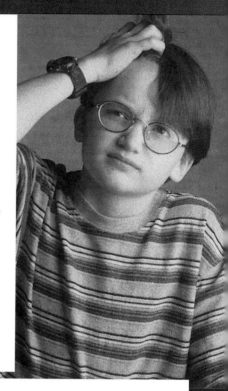

Suppose you feel stress. Ask yourself three questions:

1. What is the stressor?
2. What can I do about the stressor?
3. How can I protect my health?

Suppose you always worry about taking tests. The cause of your stress might be your desire to get high grades. Perhaps you do not study enough. If this is the case, you can do something about the cause of stress. You can spend enough time studying so that you feel prepared. You can talk to your parents about the pressure you feel to get high grades. They can help you understand that doing your best is as important as getting high grades. This can help you worry less.

Stress management skills are ways to reduce harmful effects of body changes caused by a stressor. The following skills help you deal with stress.

- **Plan your time well.** When you plan well, you are able to complete your tasks. You feel less pressure.

- **Talk to a parent, guardian, or other trusted adult.** This person can help you decide the cause of your stress and what healthful action you might take. It helps to know that others care about you.

- **Spend time with friends.** It helps to share your feelings with others who care about you.

- **Get plenty of physical activity.** Physical activity eases muscle tension. Because physical activity is fun, you can relax.

- **Eat a healthful, well-balanced diet.**

- **Stay away from foods and drinks that contain caffeine.** Caffeine is a drug that increases heart rate and blood pressure. Caffeine can keep you awake when you need sleep.

- **Write about the cause of your stress in a journal.** Health experts say this causes positive changes in your body.

Follow a...
Health Behavior Contract

Name: _____ **Date:** _____

Copy the health behavior contract on a separate sheet of paper.

DO NOT WRITE IN THIS BOOK.

Life Skill: I will have a plan for stress.

Effect on My Health: Day-to-day stressors add up and can cause health problems and disease. Some examples are headaches, stomachaches, and allergic reactions. Others are cancer and heart disease. Stress management skills are ways to reduce the effects of body changes caused by stressors. If I practice stress management skills, I will protect my health.

My Plan: I will get a notebook in which I can keep a journal. Each day for one week I will write about the stressors I experience. I will tell what I can do about each stressor. I will tell two stress management skills I used that day.

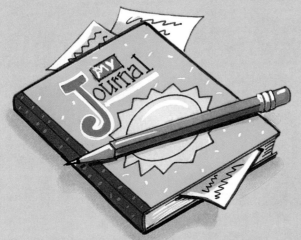

How My Plan Worked: At the end of one week, I will write a paragraph. I will tell which stressors bother me the most. I will tell which stress management skills work best for me. I will say how writing in a journal worked for me.

How Can I Bounce Back from Hard Times?

There is a saying, "Life is not fair." There is truth to this saying. Bad things can happen to very good people. For example, someone your age might follow safety guidelines at all times. This person might be crossing the street when the driver of an automobile ignores a red light. The person did nothing to cause the accident. Someone else your age might be having hard times at home. The company his or her parent worked for might have downsized. The parent could have lost his or her job and the family could be on a very tight budget. Many people your age face hard times. What can you do if you face hard times?

Keep a positive attitude. Suppose you have an eight ounce glass with four ounces of water in it. How would you describe the glass and the water? Would you describe the glass as being half-full of water? Or would you describe the glass as being half-empty?

A **positive attitude** is a positive way of thinking and seeing things. You must keep a positive attitude when there are hard times. You must focus on the glass being half-full instead of half-empty. In other words, you must focus on what is there, not what is gone or what you are without.

Depend on your support network. Your **support network** is the group of people who care about you. Members of your family and your friends make up your support network. Turn to your support network for comfort. Ask for help and understanding. During hard times, do not stay away from others. Do not feel you have to work out things without the help of others.

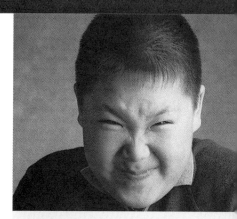

You might have done nothing to deserve hard times. But remember, you can control how you respond to hard times.

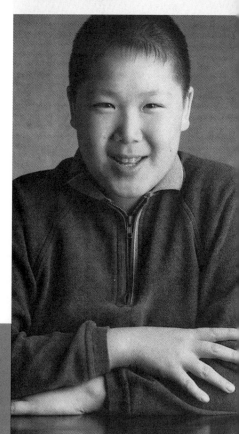

Protect your health. Hard times are stressful. They can produce distress. Practice stress management skills to reduce the harmful effects of body changes.

Do not use risk behaviors to cope. Do not turn to risk behaviors during hard times. For example, do not try to forget your troubles by drinking alcohol. Drinking alcohol harms health, is illegal, and causes more problems. Pigging out on food will not help either. You will gain weight. Getting into fights is unwise, too. You and others can become injured. Focus on choosing healthful behaviors. Then you will keep your self-respect. Others will respect you when you do not use risk behaviors to cope with hard times.

Research Update

Some physicians have studied children who experienced the death of a parent. The results from blood tests showed that the immune system of these children did not work as well after this major stressor. The physicians had the children keep a journal for several weeks. The children wrote about the death of their parent. They wrote about their feelings. Then blood samples were taken again. Writing in their journals gave their immune systems a "jump start."

Lesson 5

Review

Vocabulary

Write a separate sentence using each of the vocabulary words listed on page 30.

Health Content

Write answers to the following:

1. What body changes occur if you get stressed out? **page 31**
2. What happens if you experience eustress? Distress? **page 31**
3. What does it mean to say, "stressors add up"? **page 31**
4. What are some stress management skills to protect your health if you get stressed out? **page 32**
5. What are ways you can bounce back from hard times? **pages 34–35**

Unit 1 Review

Health Content

Review your answers for each Lesson Review in this unit. Write answers to the following questions.

1. What words are used to describe the opposite ends of *The Wellness Scale?* **Lesson 1 page 5**

2. What might you do to start the new habit of practicing a life skill? **Lesson 1 page 10**

3. How can you be sure you are making a responsible decision? **Lesson 2 page 13**

4. When should you use resistance skills? **Lesson 2 page 14**

5. What should you do if you make a mistake and do something wrong? **Lesson 3 page 17**

6. How can you show others that you are grateful? **Lesson 3 page 19**

7. What are four questions you can ask to help manage your emotions? **Lesson 4 page 24**

8. How might keeping angry feelings bottled up inside affect your health? **Lesson 4 page 25**

9. Why is it risky to get stressed out often? **Lesson 5 page 31**

10. How can having a support network help in hard times? **Lesson 5 page 34**

Guidelines for Making Responsible Decisions™

You walk over to your friend's house after school. Your friend thought you were going to ride bicycles. Since you did not bring your bicycle, your friend says you can ride double. Your friend promises to be careful. Use a separate sheet of paper. Answer "yes" or "no" to each of the following questions. Explain each answer.

1. Is it healthful for you to ride double?
2. Is it safe for you to ride double?
3. Do you follow rules and laws if you ride double?
4. Do you show respect for yourself and others if you ride double?
5. Do you follow your family's guidelines if you ride double?
6. Do you show good character if you ride double?

What is the responsible decision to make?

Family Involvement

Ask your parents or guardian to tell you five guidelines they want you to follow. Discuss each guideline. Does the guideline keep you healthy? Safe?

Vocabulary

Number a sheet of paper from 1–10. Read each definition. Next to each number on your sheet of paper, write the vocabulary word that matches the definition.

good character	mind-body connection
risk behavior	wellness
support network	responsible decision
wrong decision	positive attitude
communication	self-respect

1. A decision that is safe, healthful, and follows laws and family guidelines. **Lesson 2**
2. The good feelings you have about yourself when you behave in responsible ways. **Lesson 3**
3. The highest level of health you can reach. **Lesson 1**
4. A positive way of thinking and seeing things. **Lesson 5**
5. An action that can be harmful to you and others. **Lesson 1**
6. The idea that your thoughts and feelings have an effect on your body. **Lesson 4**
7. The group of people who care about you. **Lesson 5**
8. A decision that is harmful, unsafe, and that breaks laws or family guidelines. **Lesson 2**
9. An exchange of information with others. **Lesson 4**
10. Telling the truth, showing respect, and being fair. **Lesson 2**

Health Literacy

Effective Communication

Draw a picture or make a graphic that shows the mind-body connection. Share your art work with the class.

Self-Directed Learning

Draw and label a *Wellness Scale.* At one end of the scale, write five risk behaviors. At the other end of the scale, write five healthful behaviors.

Critical Thinking

Consider the mind-body connection. Why might having a positive attitude help keep your body healthy?

Responsible Citizenship

On an index card, write the names of three people who are part of your support network. Keep the card with you for a week. Tell the three people you are glad they are in your support network.

Multicultural Health

The word "wellness" is used in this country to mean good health. Get permission to use the computer. Find out if this word is used in other countries. How is it defined?

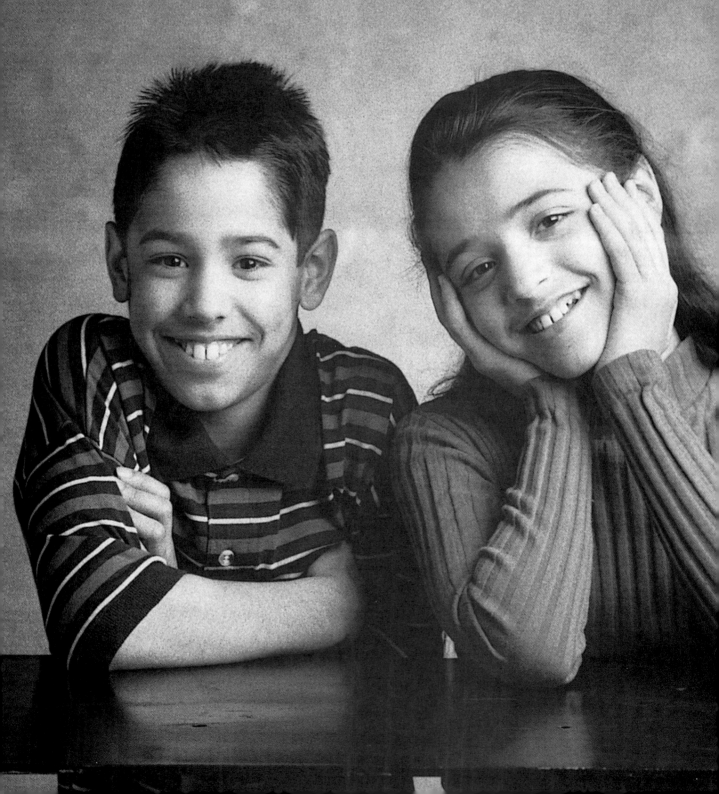

Unit 2

Family and Social Health

A Close Look at Relationships

Vocabulary

relationships: the connections you have with other people.

respect: thinking highly of someone.

honest talk: the open sharing of feelings.

mutual respect: the high regard two people have for one other.

role model: a person whose behavior other people copy.

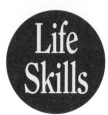

- **I will show respect for all people.**
- **I will encourage other people to take responsibility for their health.**

You come into contact with many different people. How do you treat the people with whom you come into contact? How do they treat you? What kind of influence do you have on other people? What kind of influence do other people have on you? Take a close look at your relationships.

The Lesson Objectives

- Talk about ways to show respect for others.
- Explain how to earn the respect of others.
- Talk about ways to encourage other people to take responsibility for their health.

How Can I Show Respect for Others?

Your **relationships** are the connections you have with other people. The most important part of a relationship is respect. **Respect** is thinking highly of someone. When you respect someone, you treat this person in kind ways. Put-downs are not allowed. Instead, your words encourage and support the other person. You are truthful, fair, and polite. You think about this person's feelings. You do not take advantage of this person. And you want the best for this person.

Part of showing respect for someone is being honest with your feelings. **Honest talk** is the open sharing of feelings. Honest talk involves sharing feelings that are easy for you to express. For example, you might hug a family member. You might let a friend know you think he or she is special. If a friend moves away, you might write the friend and say you miss him or her.

There are times when you need to share feelings with which you are not as comfortable. Someone you know might have a death or divorce in the family. Sharing thoughts and feelings might be difficult for you. But this is part of having a respectful relationship. If you are lost for words, you can say so. You can say, "I am sorry. I do not know what to say. I feel awkward right now." Then you show your respect for the person.

Using good manners is a way to show respect for others. Give your full attention to someone who is speaking to you. Do not interrupt or look away. If you do not understand, ask the person questions about what he or she said. Show your genuine interest.

Respect for Differences

In some ways, people have differences. They might speak a different language. They might have a different hair or skin color. They might have different beliefs. They might have special needs such as needing a wheelchair to get around. But all people want to be treated with respect. Follow the four guidelines for showing respect for people who are different from you.

- Do not tell jokes about people who are different from you.
- Do not laugh at jokes about people who are different from you.
- Do not call people who are different from you unkind names.
- Ask others not to treat people who are different from you in unkind ways.

Respect: Staying in Line

Activity

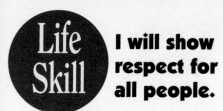

Life Skill
I will show respect for all people.

Materials: Compact disc and player or cassette and cassette recorder; space outside or in the gym

Directions: Complete the activity to learn why you need to stay in line.

1. **Read through the directions for the line dance.**
2. **Practice the steps for the line dance with your classmates.**
3. **Play music and perform the line dance.**
4. **Discuss the following questions with your classmates.**
   - Were all classmates able to "stay in line"? Why or why not?
   - Is the dance more fun if all classmates "stay in line"? Why or why not?
   - How did you feel if you got out of line? Why?
5. **Name actions that you believe are "out of line" or do not show respect for others.**

Line Dance

The following line dance is the Electric Slide. "Step" means to put your weight on a foot. "Touch" means to touch your foot on the floor, but not to put your weight on it.

1. **Step right with your right foot.** Cross your right foot behind your left foot and step with your right foot. Step left with your left foot. Touch your right foot next to your left foot.

2. **Step left with your left foot.** Cross your right foot behind your left foot and step right with your left foot. Touch your right foot next to your left foot.

3. **Step back with your right foot.** Step back with your left foot. Step back with your right foot. Touch your left heel next to your right foot.

4. **Lean forward on your left foot.** Touch your right foot behind your left foot. Lean backward on your right foot. Touch your left foot in front of your right foot.

5. **Step left with your left foot.** Turn left one-quarter turn on your left foot. Touch your right foot next to your left foot.

6. **Repeat.**

How Can I Earn the Respect of Others?

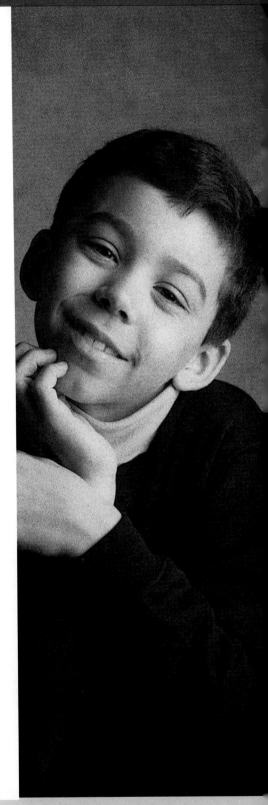

How do other people treat you? Do they treat you with respect? There are ways you can earn the respect of others.

Choose responsible behavior. Other people will have a high regard for you when you behave in responsible ways.

Treat others with respect. One way to earn the respect of others is to give respect. When you give respect, you often get respect back. **Mutual** (MYOO·chuh·wuhl) **respect** is the high regard two people have for one another. When there is mutual respect, a relationship has a balance of power. You and the other person are both important. Neither one of you pushes the other around. You take turns choosing things to do and pleasing one another. Neither one of you gets most of the attention. Both of you talk and both of you listen.

Expect others to treat you with respect. There is a saying, "Other people treat you the way you expect to be treated." Show self-respect. Do not let others treat you like a doormat. Do not let others take advantage of you or put you down. If someone does not treat you with respect, tell the person you do not want to be treated badly. For example, suppose a friend shares a secret. Tell your friend you do not appreciate his or her actions. If a friend puts you down, speak up and say something. Do not try to get even. Instead, share your feelings using an I-message.

Know when to draw the line. Suppose a person does not show respect for you even after you have talked to the person. Sometimes you need to draw the line. You need to stay away from certain people. You need to end friendships that do not have mutual respect.

How Can I Encourage Other People to Take Responsibility for Their Health?

You can encourage other people to take responsibility for their health. The most important way is to be a role model for healthful behavior. A **role model** is a person whose behavior other people copy. You can encourage others by practicing healthful behaviors yourself. Other people will see your healthful behavior. They might choose to copy it. For example, your friends might notice that you get plenty of physical activity each day. Then they might copy you and participate in physical activity.

You can talk to others about healthful behaviors. For example, you might notice that a friend skips lunch. You might encourage your friend to eat a healthful lunch. You might suggest healthful foods you know your friend enjoys.

You can support others who are trying to develop the habit of practicing a new life skill. Suppose your mother is trying to lose five pounds. You could give up eating desserts in front of her. Then she might not want to eat desserts. You could tell her that you support her. You could praise her as she loses weight.

You can share with others the efforts you make to practice life skills. For example, you might not have been getting enough sleep. You might have worked to get more sleep. You might have listened to music and taken a warm bath before bedtime. It is helpful to share your struggles and successes with others. Then other people do not think you are trying to be one up on them. They know you are working to take responsibility for your health. They are more honest with you about their struggles and successes.

Share a Health Behavior Contract

You can help another person make a health behavior contract for a life skill. First, share a health behavior contract you have made. Then help the person write out the four steps to make a health behavior contract. Offer to review the progress the person makes.

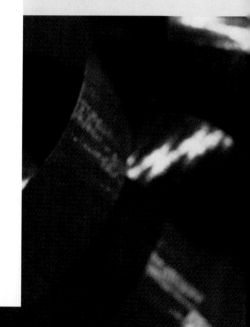

Partners in Health

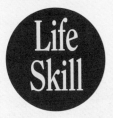

I will encourage other people to take responsibility for their health.

Materials: A partner or partners

Directions: People need people. We all need the support of other people. Follow the steps to learn the importance of support.

1. **Select a life skill from the list on pages 8–9.** The life skill should be one of interest to you.

2. **Form a partnership with one or more classmates who selected the same life skill as you did.** Discuss reasons why you selected the life skill.

3. **Make a list of ways that you could help one another make this life skill a new habit.**

Activity

Lesson 6

Review

Vocabulary

Write a separate sentence using each of the vocabulary words listed on page 40.

Health Content

Write answers to the following:

1. What are ways you can show respect for others? **page 41**

2. What are four guidelines for showing respect for people who are different from you? **page 41**

3. What are four ways to earn the respect of others? **page 43**

4. How can you encourage other people to take responsibility for their health? **page 44**

5. How does a role model help someone take responsibility for health? **page 44**

Making Peace

Vocabulary

conflict: a disagreement.

peace: being without unsettled conflicts within yourself or with others.

violence: an act that harms oneself, others, or property.

productive argument: a discussion of different viewpoints without fighting.

conflict resolution skills: steps you can take to settle disagreements in a responsible way.

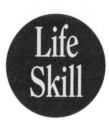

Life Skill

• **I will settle conflict in healthful ways.**

Throughout life you will experience conflicts. A **conflict** is a disagreement. You might have a conflict within yourself. You might have to make a choice between two things. Maybe you are pulled in two directions. You might have a conflict with another person. The two of you see things in a different way. A conflict needs to be settled. How will you settle a conflict?

The Lesson Objectives

● Explain how settling internal conflict protects your health.

● Explain how settling conflict with others protects your health.

● List and discuss ways to settle conflicts.

How Does Settling Conflicts Within Myself and with Others Protect My Health?

Peace is being without unsettled conflicts within yourself or with others. Settling conflicts within yourself and with others protects your health. Suppose you do not have conflicts within yourself. Then you are not pulled in two different directions. You are less likely to be anxious and upset. You are less likely to experience the body changes from being stressed out. As a result, you are better able to sleep. You are less likely to get health conditions such as headaches and upset stomach. You are even less likely to have rashes and allergies. If you are at peace with yourself, you are more likely to live a longer and healthier life.

Suppose you settle conflicts with others. This protects your health, too. Being at peace with others improves relationships. Other people know you are not trying to pick a fight. They know they can be honest with you. This is because you will work things out. You will be calm and show respect. You are more likely to have close friends.

Being able to settle conflicts helps reduce the risk of harm from violence. **Violence** is an act that harms oneself, others, or property. If you get into fights, you can get injured. You can get bruises, cuts, scrapes, or a black eye. You can get a knocked out tooth or broken bones. Suppose you fight with someone who has a weapon. This person might use the weapon to harm you. A gunshot can cause blindness, paralysis, and death. You protect yourself from injury when you know how to settle conflict.

Productive Arguments Versus Fighting

Everyone has arguments. But an argument should not lead to a fight. Instead, it should be productive. A **productive argument** is a discussion of different viewpoints without fighting.

A peaceful solution must result in actions that:

- are healthful;
- are safe;
- follow rules and laws;
- follow your family's guidelines;
- show respect for you and others;
- show good character.

How Can I Settle Conflicts Without Fighting?

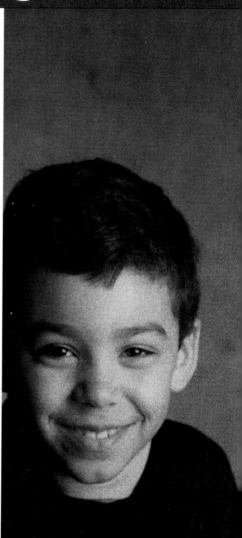

Conflict resolution skills are steps you can take to settle disagreements in a responsible way.

1. **Remain calm.**
2. **Set the tone.**
    - Do not blame.
    - Do not interrupt.
    - Do not use put-downs.
3. **Talk about what happened.**
4. **Be honest about what you have said or done to cause the disagreement.**
5. **Use I-messages to express your feelings about what happened.**
6. **Listen to the feelings of the other person.**
7. **List and talk about possible solutions.** Ask:
    - Will the solution lead to actions that are healthful?
    - Will the solution lead to actions that are safe?
    - Will the solution lead to actions that follow rules and laws?
    - Will the solution lead to actions that show respect for you and others?
    - Will the solution lead to actions that follow your family's guidelines?
    - Will the solution lead to actions that show you have good character?
8. **Agree on a solution.**
9. **Keep your word and follow the solution upon which you agreed.**
10. **Ask a trusted adult for help if you cannot agree to a solution.**

Use... Guidelines for Making Responsible Decisions™

You are playing softball with classmates. The pitcher throws a ball that hits the batter who is on your team. During the next inning, the opposing pitcher will be up to bat. You are the pitcher for your team. Your teammates want you to throw a ball that hits the pitcher. They want to get even.

?

Use a separate sheet of paper. Answer "yes" or "no" to each of the following questions. Explain each answer.

1. Is it healthful for you to throw a ball that hits the pitcher?
2. Is it safe for you to throw a ball that hits the pitcher?
3. Do you follow rules and laws if you throw a ball that hits the pitcher?
4. Do you show respect for yourself and others if you throw a ball that hits the pitcher?
5. Do you follow your family's guidelines if you throw a ball that hits the pitcher?
6. Do you show good character if you throw a ball that hits the pitcher?

What is the responsible decision to make?

Lesson 7

Review

Vocabulary

Write a separate sentence using each of the vocabulary words listed on page 46.

Health Content

Write answers to the following:

1. How does settling conflict within yourself protect your health? **page 47**
2. How does settling conflict with others protect your health? **page 47**
3. How do you know if a solution is a peaceful one? **page 47**
4. What are ten steps you can take to settle disagreements? **page 48**
5. What are three suggestions for setting the tone before talking about conflict? **page 48**

What Counts in Friendship

Vocabulary

bonding: a process in which two people develop feelings of closeness for one other.

social skills: skills that help you interact with others.

clique: a group of people who keep other people out of their group.

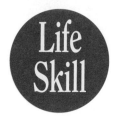

• I will work to have healthful friendships.

A friend is someone you know well and like. A friend is someone with whom you can share fun activities. When you need support and encouragement, you can turn to a friend. Do you invest time and energy in your friendships?

The Lesson Objectives

● Discuss reasons why you need friends.

● List and discuss guidelines for friendships.

● Discuss reasons to avoid being in a clique.

Why Do I Need Friends?

Bonding is a process in which two people develop feelings of closeness for one another. The ties of friendship improve the quality of your life.

When you have close friends, you do not feel lonely. You have friends with whom you can share thoughts, feelings, and activities.

Friends can help you develop other parts of your personality. They can encourage you to learn new skills. They can show interest in your talents and hobbies. When you spend time with friends, you learn about yourself. You improve your social skills. **Social skills** are skills that help you interact with others.

Throughout life you might experience hard times. Friends are part of your support network. They are there to support and encourage you during hard times. No matter how hard times are, you have your friends.

Having close friendships improves physical health. Health experts know that people who have close friendships have better health. Being cared about causes healthful changes inside your body. When you feel cared about, your body is better able to fight disease. This is because the body changes caused by stressors do not last as long.

Animals can be good friends, too. Health experts say that people who have a pet enjoy some health benefits. Suppose you feel stressed. Your pet might greet you when you return home. You might talk to your pet. You might take your pet for a walk. Petting and caring for an animal can help lower stress.

Feedback from Your Parents or Guardian

Your parents or guardian probably tell you what they think of your friends. They know that friends can influence you. They want you to choose friends that are responsible. They want you to choose friends who have good character.

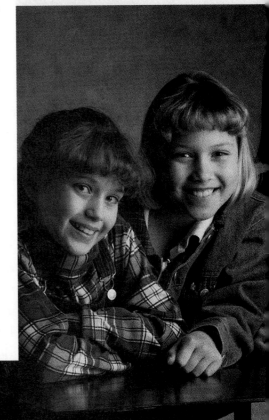

What Are Guidelines for Friendships?

Use the following guidelines for friendship. These guidelines strengthen the bonds of friendship. They help you have responsible and healthful friendships.

Make responsible decisions with friends. Use the *Guidelines for Making Responsible Decisions™*. Do not give in to peer pressure to make wrong decisions. If you go along with wrong decisions, you will not keep your self-respect. Even the friends who pressure you will lose respect for you.

Talk over your disagreements. You can disagree with someone and still be friends. Find a private place to talk. Use the conflict resolution skills that are in Lesson 7. Working through disagreements can make the ties of friendship stronger.

Keep promises that you make. Think before you make a promise. Be certain that you check out your family responsibilities before making promises. After you make a promise, your friend depends on you. Being dependable is very important in a friendship.

Encourage each other to grow. A healthful friendship promotes growth. When you are with a friend, think of new activities to enjoy. Do not get into a rut and do the same thing all the time.

Keep confidences. Trust is an important part of friendship. Do not share what a friend tells you in confidence.

Allow each other time to be alone and time for family members and other friends. It is not healthful to spend all your time with the same friend. You and a friend need time alone to think and be in touch with feelings. You need time for family members and other friends.

When a Friend Needs Help

Suppose a friend tells you he or she is doing or going to do something wrong. For example, you might find out that the friend is using drugs or stealing. These actions are harmful and illegal. Do not keep these actions secret. Tell a responsible adult right away. Your friend needs help. Your actions protect your friend.

Why Should I Avoid Being in a Clique?

A **clique** (CLIK) is a group of people who keep other people out of their group. Suppose five classmates hang out together. They do everything together and do not want others to join them. For example, these five classmates might eat lunch together. If another classmate tries to join them, they might ignore him or her.

You and others who are your age want to feel like you belong. There is a need to feel accepted and important. But leaving others out is not the best way to gain these feelings. How would you feel if you could not join others when you wanted to? How would you feel if others ignored you when you were around?

Social skills help you interact with others. Being in a clique can keep you from developing social skills. You will not have the opportunity to interact with different kinds of people. People who are different from you can give you new ideas. They can improve your thinking. If you are in a clique, you will not gain skills in making new friends. As you get older, you will regret that you did not interact with a wide range of people. These interactions not only improve social skills, they help you gain self-confidence in social situations.

There is another reason to avoid being in a clique. If you are in a clique, you are more likely to do the same things. You are more likely to discuss the same things again and again. Suppose you have a variety of friends. Your friends will have different interests and skills. They will expose you to new interests and skills. As a result, you will be a more interesting person. People tend to like a person who gets along with a wide range of people. People tend to like a person who has many interests and skills.

Say YES to Social Skills–Say NO to Cliques

- **Include new people in your group of friends.**
- **Go out of your way to meet people who are not in your group of friends.**
- **Say NO if your group of friends wants to leave out others for no good reason.**

Follow a...
Health Behavior Contract

Name:_____ **Date:**_____

Life Skill: I will work to have healthful friendships.

Effect on My Health: Having healthful friendships improves health. I will practice and improve my social skills. I will enjoy healthful activities with friends. I will not feel lonely. Health experts say that having close friends reduces the effects of stress.

My Plan: I want to make sure that I follow the guidelines for friendship. I am going to keep a Friendship Diary for one week. Each night, I will write about one of my friendships. I will answer the following questions.

1. Did I make responsible decisions with my friend?
2. If we had a disagreement, did we talk it over?
3. Did I promise I would do something? Did I keep my promise?
4. Did we do something new? Do we always do the same thing?
5. Can my friend trust me to keep secrets?
6. Did I allow my friend time to be with others?

How My Plan Worked: At the end of the week, I will read my Friendship Diary. I will rate how well I followed the guidelines for friendship.

Use... Guidelines for Making Responsible Decisions™

Your teacher introduces a new classmate. The new classmate has just moved into your neighborhood. You have plans to eat lunch with your group of friends. The new classmate wants to join you. One of your friends says, "Don't let that nerd spoil our group."

Use a separate sheet of paper. Answer "yes" or "no" to each of the following questions. Explain each answer.

1. Is it healthful for you to exclude the new classmate?
2. Is it safe for you to exclude the new classmate?
3. Do you follow rules and laws if you exclude the new classmate?
4. Do you show respect for yourself and others if you exclude the new classmate?
5. Do you follow your family's guidelines if you exclude the new classmate?
6. Do you show good character if you exclude the new classmate?

What is the responsible decision to make?

Lesson 8
Review

Vocabulary

Write a separate sentence using each of the vocabulary words listed on page 50.

Health Content
Write answers to the following:

1. Why do you need friends? **page 51**
2. What are six guidelines for friendship? **page 52**
3. When should you to talk to an adult about a secret a friend has told you? **page 52**
4. Why should you avoid being in a clique? **page 53**
5. How can you say YES to social skills and NO to cliques? **page 53**

The Family Bond

Vocabulary

family: the group of people to whom you are related.

family guideline: a rule set by your parents or guardian that helps you know how to act.

character: the effort you use to act on responsible values.

heredity: the traits that you get from your natural parents.

habit: a usual way of doing something.

family value: the worth or importance of something to your family.

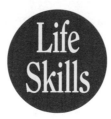

Life Skills

- **I will work to have healthful family relationships.**
- **I will adjust to family changes in healthful ways.**

Your **family** is the group of people to whom you are related. Your relationships with family members are important. *Bonding* is a process in which two people develop feelings of closeness for one another. When you bond with members of your family, you feel you are loved. You feel like you belong.

The Lesson Objectives

- Explain why you need to follow family guidelines.
- Discuss ways your family influences your health.
- List and discuss changes that occur in some families.

Why Do I Need to Follow Family Guidelines?

Your family has guidelines for you to follow. A **family guideline** is a rule set by your parents or guardian that helps you know how to act. There are reasons why your parents or guardian have set family guidelines. And there are reasons why you should follow them.

Family guidelines protect you.

When you follow family guidelines, you protect:

- your health;
- your safety;
- the laws of the community.

For example, your parents or guardian might expect you to answer the telephone a certain way if they are not home. They might tell you what to do if a stranger comes to your door. They might have set family guidelines to follow in case of fire. These family guidelines protect your safety.

Family guidelines make sure you show respect for other family members.

Your parents or guardians teach you how to show respect. They expect you to use manners. They expect you to settle disagreements without fighting or put-downs. Then you can apply these actions to other relationships. You show respect for others.

Family guidelines teach you about good character.

Character is the effort you use to act on responsible values. Your parents or guardians share their values. Then they expect you to follow through and show these values. For example, they might value your health. As a result, they expect you not to drink alcohol or try other drugs. This is how you learn good character.

Family Guidelines Are a Sign of Love

Love is both a feeling and an action. A parent or guardian can have loving feelings for children. But a parent or guardian must have loving actions, too. Loving actions include taking steps to protect children. This is why a loving parent or guardian sets family guidelines. And this is why a loving parent or guardian corrects you if you break a family guideline.

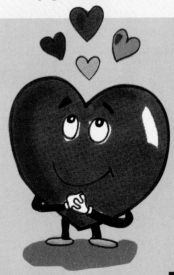

How Does My Family Influence My Health?

Your *lifestyle* is your way of living. Your lifestyle includes the habits you choose. It includes the environment in which you live. Your lifestyle includes the kinds of relationships you have. It includes the guidelines and values that are important to you. Your family influences your lifestyle. This is how your family influences your health.

Family heredity influences your health.

Heredity is the traits that you get from your natural parents. Some traits are your height, skin color, and chances of having certain diseases. Think about some of the diseases that are influenced by heredity. For example, some kinds of heart disease and cancer occur more often in some families. A natural parent or grandparent might have high blood pressure. This would raise your risk of having high blood pressure. A natural parent or grandparent might have had colon cancer. Colon cancer occurs more often in some families.

Of course, heredity only raises the risk. There are actions you can take to lower the risk of having a disease that runs in your family.

Suppose high blood pressure runs in your family. You can take actions to lower the risk of having high blood pressure. You can stay at a healthful weight. You can keep arteries clear by eating a low-fat diet. You can get plenty of physical activity. Suppose colon cancer runs in your family. You can take actions to lower the risk of having colon cancer. You can get plenty of physical activity. Your diet can include plenty of fiber, such as cereal, fruits, and vegetables. These foods help you have a daily bowel movement.

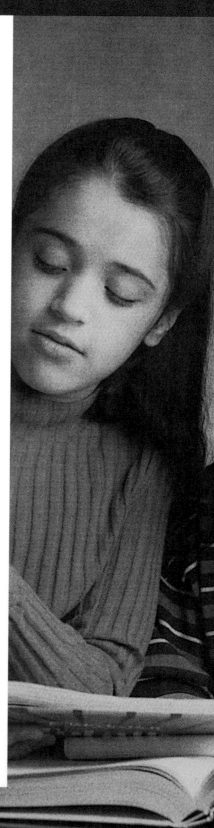

Family habits influence your health.

A **habit** is a usual way of doing something. Suppose your family eats low-fat foods and limits salt. Then you are more likely to develop these eating habits. Suppose your parent or guardian gets plenty of physical activity. Then you are more likely to participate in physical activity. But suppose your parent or guardian is a couch potato and eats junk foods. You might make these risk behaviors a habit.

Family environment influences your health.

Your *environment* is everything that is around you. Suppose your family lives near the mountains. You might learn to ski, snowboard, or mountain climb. You can take part in these physical activities in this environment. Suppose you live in a crowded area. Perhaps there is much noise where you live. Then you must cope with being crowded and having noise. Some young people live in neighborhoods where there is much crime and violence. These young people must work extra hard to protect their safety.

Family relationships influence your health.

The quality of family relationships is known to have an important influence on health. Health experts have studied the effects of bonding on behavior. Suppose you feel close to members of your family. Health experts say you are more likely to avoid risk behaviors. This is because you feel loved and accepted by the important people in your life. You know they will support you.

Some young people do not feel close to members of their families. Health experts say they are more likely to choose risk behaviors. This is because they look for love and acceptance outside their families. They are more easily influenced by their peers. They might do what peers say to feel like they belong.

Family guidelines and values influence your health.

A **family value** is the worth or importance of something to your family. You are more likely to choose healthful behaviors if your family places a value on good health. You are more likely to choose healthful behaviors if family guidelines encourage you to do so.

What Are Changes That Occur in Some Families?

Family size increases with a birth, adoption, or foster child.

Changes occur when there is a new family member. A baby might be born. A baby or child might be adopted. To *adopt* is to take a child of other parents into your family. A foster child might come to live with you. A *foster child* is a child who lives in a family without being related by birth or adoption. Other children in the family might have new responsibilites. They might have feelings about the changes that occur. For example, they might get less attention at first. Family members can share feelings with each other as they learn to adjust.

A family member is ill.

Perhaps a grandparent becomes ill and needs care. If the grandparent lives with the family, family members pitch in and help. If the family member is in the hospital, parents might be gone more. When changes are brought about by illness, cooperation is important.

Parents get separated or divorced.

Usually parents can solve problems in their marriage. But sometimes they cannot. A *separation* is a situation in which parents are married but living apart. During this time, some parents solve their problems and live together again.

Sometimes parents are unable to solve their problems. A *divorce* is a legal way to end a marriage. Divorce can be very hard for children. Children might feel insecure and very sad. They might feel guilty although they are not to blame. Talking helps children and their parents understand each other's feelings.

Use... Guidelines for Making Responsible Decisions™

Your parent or guardian is at a neighbor's house. They ask you to keep the door locked and not to answer it when they are not home. A stranger comes to your door. The stranger says he has a present for your parent or guardian. The stranger asks you to open the door to sign for the present.

Use a separate sheet of paper. Answer "yes" or "no" to each of the following questions. Explain each answer.

1. Is it healthful for you to open the door to the stranger?

2. Is it safe for you to open the door to the stranger?

3. Do you follow rules and laws if you open the door to the stranger?

4. Do you show respect for yourself and others if you open the door to the stranger?

5. Do you follow your family's guidelines if you open the door to the stranger?

6. Do you show good character if you open the door to the stranger?

What is the responsible decision to make?

Lesson 9

Review

Vocabulary

Write a separate sentence using each of the vocabulary words listed on page 56.

Health Content

Write answers to the following:

1. What are three reasons why you need to follow family guidelines? **page 57**

2. Why does a loving parent or guardian correct you if you break a family guideline? **page 57**

3. What are five ways your family influences your health? **pages 58–59**

4. Why are you more likely to choose healthful behaviors if you are close to your family? **page 59**

5. What three changes can occur in families? **page 60**

Abstinence Now Protects My Future

Vocabulary

abstinence: choosing not to be sexually active.

reputation: the quality of your character as judged by others.

guilt: the bad feelings you have if you think or do something that you know is not right.

marriage: a legal commitment that a couple makes to love and care for one another.

resistance skills: skills that help you resist pressure to make a wrong decision.

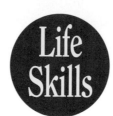

Life Skills

- **I will prepare for future relationships.**
- **I will practice abstinence.**

Suppose you have a test in a week. To prepare for the test, you plan now to study every day. You begin by studying for an hour right now. On the day of the test, your plan pays off. You are ready for the test. In the same way, you need to plan right now for future relationships. If you do, your plan will pay off. You will benefit from your efforts.

The Lesson Objectives

- Explain why you are learning about abstinence.
- List and discuss reasons to choose abstinence.
- List and discuss skills that help you practice abstinence.

Why Am I Learning About Abstinence?

Abstinence (AB·stuh·nuhnts) is choosing not to be sexually active. You might wonder why you are learning about abstinence. You might think, "I can talk about this when I am older." But you need to prepare for your future right now. There is good reason for you to discuss abstinence with your parents or guardian right now. They want you to know why abstinence is important. They want to protect you. Your parents or guardian want to guide you so that you are responsible.

You can avoid making a mistake for which there will be serious outcomes.

Your parents or guardian probably have talked to you about drinking alcohol. They want you to know what to do in certain situations. They give you guidelines to protect you. For example, they tell you what to do if someone offers you a ride home who has been drinking. They tell you to call them. They do not want you to get into a car with someone who drives after drinking alcohol. You know their guideline protects you. You do not want to be injured or die in a crash. In this lesson, you will learn facts about abstinence. You will learn why your parents or guardian want you to practice abstinence. You will learn the serious outcomes that can occur when young people do not practice abstinence.

You need to have skills to help you practice abstinence.

You need to be ready if someone tries to get you to change your mind about abstinence. You do not want to be taken off guard. This means you should learn skills now. You need to learn how to say NO to pressure. You cannot wait until you are in a situation to learn these skills.

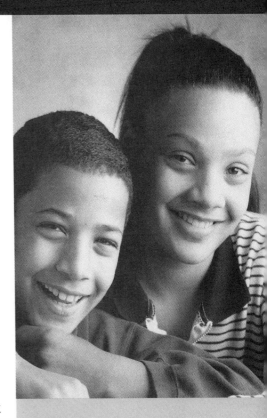

Follow Family Guidelines

Why Should I Choose Abstinence?

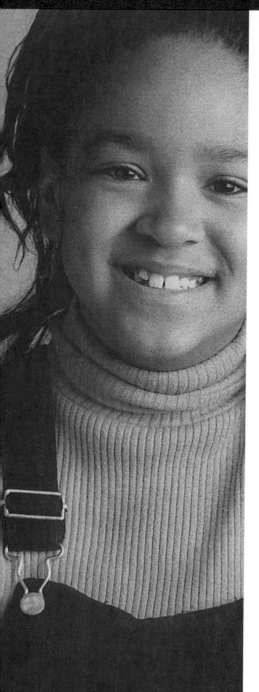

Suppose you were asked to give reasons why abstinence is best for you. There are ten reasons you can give. Read through the ten reasons below. You will see why you make a responsible decision when you choose abstinence. You show respect for the guidelines of your parents or guardian. You stay healthy. You keep your self-respect. You show good character.

1. **I want to follow family guidelines.** My parents or guardian want me to practice abstinence. They want me to protect my future. I want to protect my future and obey them.

2. **I want to respect myself.** I want to be very special. I do not want someone to use me or talk me into something I do not want to do.

3. **I want to respect others.** I want to show others that I think well of them. I do not want to use someone or talk someone into disobeying their parent or guardian.

4. **I want to have a good reputation. Reputation** is the quality of your character as judged by others. I want others to believe I have responsible values.

5. **I do not want to feel guilty. Guilt** is the bad feelings you have if you think or do something that you know is not right. I want to have positive feelings. I want to sleep at night knowing I am doing what I believe to be right.

6. **I am not ready for marriage.** A **marriage** is a legal commitment that a couple makes to love and care for one another. I do not have the skills, education, or money I need to make this commitment right now.

7. **I do not want to risk pregnancy.** (Females) My body is not ready for a pregnancy. I am growing and developing. If I got pregnant, I would risk my health and the health of the baby. (Males) I do not want to get someone pregnant. I would not want her to risk her health. I would not want to risk the health of the baby.

8. **I am not ready to be a parent.** Being a parent requires a commitment of my time, skills, and money. I am busy with school and preparing for my future. I am still learning skills such as how a baby learns and develops. I have not finished school and cannot get a job that could pay me enough to be married and raise a child.

9. **I do not want to be infected with an STD.** A *sexually transmitted disease*, or *STD*, is a disease caused by pathogens that are spread during sexual contact. If I have sex, the person I have sex with might have an STD. The person might not tell me. Or the person might not even know he or she has an STD. This is too risky. There is no cure for some STDs.

10. **I do not want to be infected with HIV.** *HIV* is the virus that destroys helper T cells and causes AIDS. If I have sex, the person I have sex with might be infected with HIV. The person might not tell me. Or the person might not even know he or she is infected with HIV. This is too risky. There is no cure for HIV and AIDS right now.

How Can I Prepare Now to Practice Abstinence?

Resistance skills are skills that help you resist pressure to make a wrong decision. At some time, a person might pressure you to change your mind about abstinence. This person wants you to disobey your family guidelines. This person wants you to risk your health. This person wants you to risk your reputation. Prepare now to resist the pressure.

1. **Say, "NO. I choose abstinence."**
2. **Give reasons for saying NO.**
   - Use one or two reasons from the list on pages 64–65.
   - Repeat the same reasons several times if necessary.
3. **Be certain your behavior matches your words.**
   - Do not lead someone on.
4. **Avoid being in a situation in which someone might pressure you to have sex.**
   - Be with several friends rather than being alone.
   - Stay away from places where pressure can take place, such as in someone's home while parents are gone.
5. **Avoid being with people who make wrong decisions.**
   - Choose friends who encourage you to choose abstinence.
   - Choose friends who do not drink alcohol.
6. **Tell an adult if you are pressured.**
   - Get support and suggestions from the adult.
7. **Encourage your friends to choose abstinence.**

Choose TV Programs Approved by Your Parents or Guardian

Peers are not the only ones who can influence you. Suppose you turn on a TV program. The teens on the program do not practice abstinence. You might begin to think this is OK if you watch the program often. Choose TV programs carefully. Look up to teens who make responsible decisions.

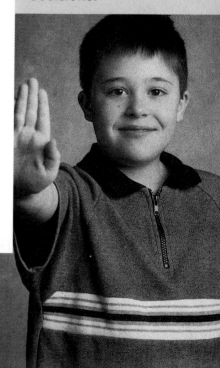

Abstinence Pledge Card

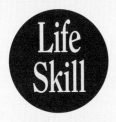

I will practice abstinence.

Materials: Index cards, pen or pencil

Directions: A pledge is a promise to do something. Complete this activity and share your pledge card with your parents or guardian.

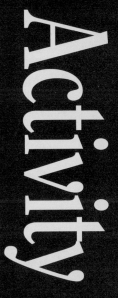

Activity

1. **Review pages 64–65.** Select several reasons you believe abstinence is important.

2. **Use the index card and design a pledge card.** Put the following information on your pledge card.
   - A heading: "I pledge to choose abstinence because..."
   - A list of at least five reasons you pledge to choose abstinence
   - Your signature
   - The date
   - A place for your parent's or guardian's signature and the date

3. **Review your pledge card with your parents or guardian.** Sign and date your pledge card.

Lesson 10

Review

Vocabulary

Write a separate sentence using each of the vocabulary words listed on page 62.

Health Content

Write answers to the following:

1. What are two reasons you are learning about abstinence? **page 63**

2. What are ten reasons why abstinence is best for you? **pages 64–65**

3. Why is it risky to get infected with STDs or HIV? **page 65**

4. What are seven resistance skills you can use to practice abstinence? **page 66**

5. How can you avoid being in a situation in which someone might try to get you to change your mind about abstinence? **page 66**

Unit 2 Review

Health Content

Review your answers for each Lesson Review in this unit. Write answers to the following questions.

1. What are four ways to show respect for people who are different from you? **Lesson 6 page 41**

2. How do you know if there is mutual respect in a relationship? **Lesson 6 page 43**

3. Why do you need to be at peace with yourself? **Lesson 7 page 47**

4. What are conflict resolution skills? **Lesson 7 page 48**

5. How might having a pet improve health? **Lesson 8 page 51**

6. Why do some young people form cliques? **Lesson 8 page 53**

7. What happens when you bond with family members? **Lesson 9 page 56**

8. Will you always develop a disease if the disease occurs in your family? **Lesson 9 page 58**

9. Why is it risky for someone your age to be pregnant? **Lesson 10 page 65**

10. Why is it risky to be infected with an STD or HIV? **Lesson 10 page 65**

Guidelines for Making Responsible Decisions™

Two of your friends do not like one of your classmates who is different from them. They call your classmate unkind names and poke fun at her. They find out your classmate's family has a computer with e-mail. They want you to send threats by e-mail to scare your classmate. They say you will not get caught. Use a separate sheet of paper. Answer "yes" or "no" to each of the following questions. Explain each answer.

1. Is it healthful to send threats by e-mail to your classmate?

2. Is it safe to send threats by e-mail to your classmate?

3. Do you follow rules and laws if you send threats by e-mail to your classmate?

4. Do you show respect for yourself and others if you send threats by e-mail to your classmate?

5. Do you follow your family's guidelines if you send threats by e-mail to your classmate?

6. Do you show good character if you send threats by e-mail to your classmate?

What is the responsible decision to make?

Vocabulary

Number a sheet of paper from 1–10. Read each definition. Next to each number on your sheet of paper, write the vocabulary word that matches the definition.

mutual respect	violence
bonding	family value
reputation	role model
peace	clique
habit	abstinence

1. The high regard two people have for one another. **Lesson 6**
2. The worth or importance of something to your family. **Lesson 9**
3. Being without unsettled conflicts within yourself or with others. **Lesson 7**
4. Choosing not to be sexually active. **Lesson 10**
5. A person whose behavior other people copy. **Lesson 6**
6. An usual way of doing something. **Lesson 9**
7. A process in which two people develop feelings of closeness for one another. **Lesson 8**
8. The quality of your character as judged by others. **Lesson 10**
9. An act that harms oneself, others, or property. **Lesson 7**
10. A group of people who keep other people out of their group. **Lesson 8**

Multicultural Health

You might show respect for your parents or guardian by finishing chores before asked. Research how young people in another culture show respect for parents or adults. Write a paragraph.

Health Literacy

Effective Communication

Sing this song in rounds with your class. "Make new friends, but keep the old. One is silver and the other gold." Discuss the meaning of this song.

Self-Directed Learning

Write a bibliography that includes information about three books on friendship. Also, include a short description of what is in each book.

Critical Thinking

Write a paragraph to answer the following question. Why do elderly people who are visited often in nursing homes have better health than those who have no visitors?

Responsible Citizenship

Decide to be a role model for a healthful behavior. Select the healthful behavior. Brainstorm three ways you can be a good role model.

Family Involvement

Work with your parents or guardian to list ten family guidelines. Make a booklet of these guidelines to keep in your home.

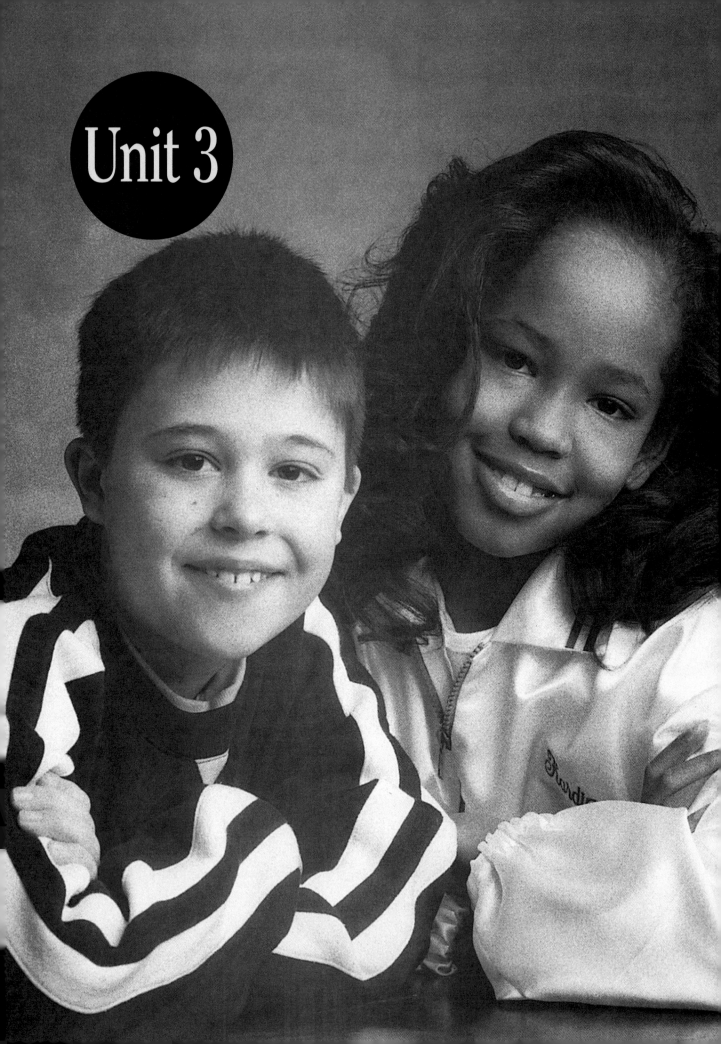

Unit 3

Growth and Development

Body Systems Review

Vocabulary

skeletal system: forms a framework to support the body and to help protect internal soft tissues.

muscular system: helps you move and maintain posture.

nervous system: the system for communication and control.

digestive system: breaks down food so that it can be used by the body.

circulatory system: transports oxygen, food, and waste through the body.

respiratory system: helps the body use the air you breathe.

endocrine system: is made up of glands.

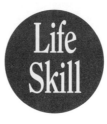
Life Skill

● **I will care for my body systems.**

Your body is made up of cells, tissues, and organs. A *cell* is the smallest living part of the body. Muscles are made up of muscle cells. A *tissue* is a group of cells that work together. For example, skin cells are flat and thin and fit tightly together. They make up skin tissue. An *organ* is a group of tissues that work together. The heart is an organ. A *body system* is a group of organs that work together to carry out certain tasks.

The Lesson Objectives

● Discuss the tasks carried out by each body system.

● Tell ways to care for each body system.

How Can I Care for My Skeletal System?

Your **skeletal system** is the body system that forms a framework to support the body and to help protect internal soft tissues. There are over 200 bones in your body. Bones have many different tasks. Your bones work with your muscles to support your body. Bones protect inner body parts. For example, your skull protects your brain.

Bone marrow (MEHR·oh) is the soft tissue in the middle of long bones. Bone marrow helps your body make thousands of red blood cells each day. Red blood cells are cells in the blood that carry oxygen to all body cells. White blood cells are made in bone marrow. White blood cells help destroy harmful organisms in the body and remove dead cells.

A *joint* is a place where two bones meet. Your joints allow your bones to move. There are different kinds of joints in your body. The joints in your shoulders allow you to move your arms in circles. The elbow joint allows you to bend your arm. Bones are connected by ligaments at joints. *Ligaments* (LIG·uh·muhnts) are bands of tissue that hold bones together at movable joints. Your knees and elbows are examples of movable joints. *Tendons* (TEN·duhnz) are tough tissue fibers that connect muscles to bones.

As you grow older, your bones continue to change. New bone cells grow at the end of your bones. Your bones continue to grow until you are about 20 years old.

- Choose foods and drinks that are a source of calcium. Examples are milk, cheese, yogurt, and low-fat ice cream. Calcium makes bones stronger.
- Get plenty of physical activity to make bones thicker and stronger.
- Follow safety guidelines to prevent injuries to bones, joints, ligaments, and tendons.

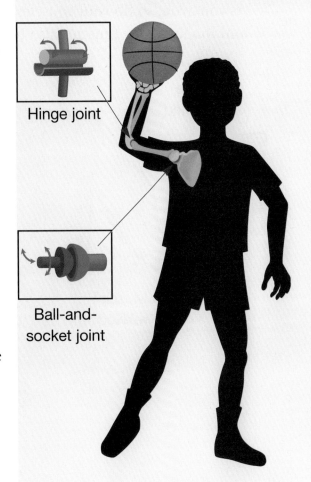

Hinge joint

Ball-and-socket joint

How Can I Care for My Muscular System?

Your **muscular system** is the body system that helps you move and maintain posture. Every movement in your body is caused by moving your muscles. Some muscles work in pairs. When one muscle in a pair contracts or shortens, the other relaxes. Your body can move because your muscles contract.

You have different kinds of muscles in your body. *Voluntary muscles* are muscles that you control. The muscles in your arm are voluntary muscles. You control how and when you move your arm. *Involuntary muscles* are muscles that work automatically. Your heart is an involuntary muscle. Your heart beats on its own. As you grow, so do your muscles. They grow thicker and longer. Your muscles also become firmer.

- Choose physical activities to strengthen different muscle groups.
- Choose physical activities that strengthen the arms, legs, and heart.
- Choose physical activities that stretch muscles.

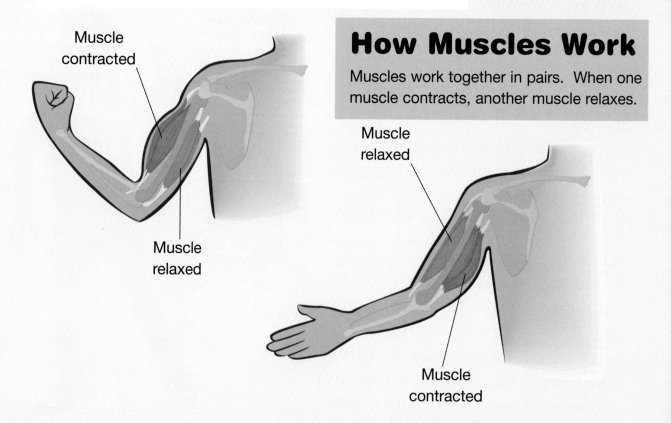

Muscle contracted

Muscle relaxed

How Muscles Work

Muscles work together in pairs. When one muscle contracts, another muscle relaxes.

Muscle relaxed

Muscle contracted

How Can I Care for My Nervous System?

Your **nervous system** is the body system for communication and control. It is made up of a network of cells. These cells send and receive messages to and from your brain and spinal cord to all parts of your body. Your nervous system includes your brain, spinal cord, and branching nerves. Your brain and spinal cord work together. Messages travel to and from branching nerves in the body. Nerve tissue is made of nerve cells called neurons (NOO·rahnz).

Suppose someone throws a ball to you. Your eyes see the ball and send a message to your brain. Your brain helps you respond to catch the ball. It sends signals to your muscles. Your muscles move so you can catch the ball.

Your brain is like a computer. It can carry out many functions. The *cerebrum* (suh·REE·bruhm) is the part of the brain that controls your ability to learn, your memory, and your voluntary muscle control. The *cerebellum* (ser·uh·BEL·uhm) is the part of the brain that controls how well your muscles work together. It helps make your movements smooth and graceful and controls your balance. Your *medulla* (muh·DUH·luh) is the part of the brain that controls actions such as heart rate and breathing.

Your *spinal cord* is a thick band of nerve cells through which messages enter and leave the brain. The spinal cord is involved in all the senses. Suppose you touch an object. Nerves throughout your body travel from the skin of your fingers to your spinal cord. The spinal cord then sends a message to the brain. You respond. What do you do when you touch ice? What do you do when you smell a carton of spoiled milk?

- Use a safety restraint system when riding in a car.
- Wear a safety helmet for sports.
- Stay away from all harmful drugs, including alcohol.
- Do not breathe toxic fumes, such as glue.

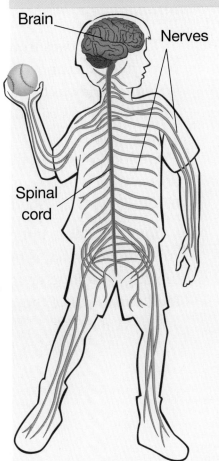

Brain

Nerves

Spinal cord

How Can I Care for My Digestive System?

Your **digestive system** is the body system that breaks down food so that it can be used by the body. Your body needs food to help it work.

Digestion is the way in which the food you eat is changed and used by your body's cells. Digestion begins in your mouth. Your teeth and saliva begin to change the food. Your tongue helps push food down the esophagus (ih·SAHF·uh·gus). The food moves into your stomach. Digestive juices in your stomach further break down the food. At this point, the food takes the form of a thick paste.

The food moves from your stomach to your small intestine. Here, digested food becomes ready to be used by your body's cells. Structures called villi (VIH·ly) line your small intestine. Villi are shaped like fingers. Tiny blood vessels in the villi absorb the digested food into your bloodstream. Your blood delivers this food to your body cells.

Your body does not digest everything you eat. Food that is not digested moves to the large intestine or colon. Undigested food passes out of the body through the anus (AY·nus).

- Chew food thoroughly to make it easier to digest.
- Eat foods that contain fiber, such as grains and fruit, to help you have a daily bowel movement.
- Drink six to eight glasses of water each day.

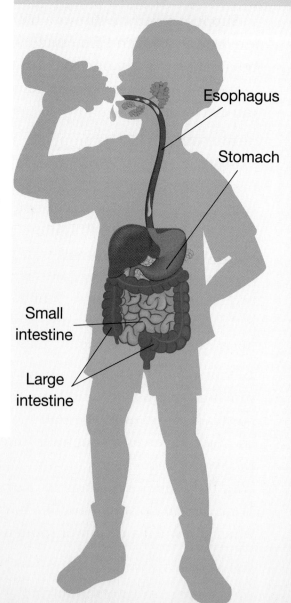

Esophagus

Stomach

Small intestine

Large intestine

How Can I Care for My Circulatory System?

Your **circulatory** (SUHR·kyuh·luh·TOR·ee) **system** is the body system that transports oxygen, food, and waste through the body. The circulatory system is made up of the heart, blood, and blood vessels.

Your heart is a muscle about the size of a closed fist. It weighs only 10 or 11 ounces. Your heart pumps blood throughout your body. Your heart muscle has four parts. It has two upper parts and two lower parts. The *atria* (AY·tree·uh) are the upper parts of the heart. The *ventricles* (VEN·tri·kuhlz) are the lower parts of the heart. Your heart has two atria and two ventricles.

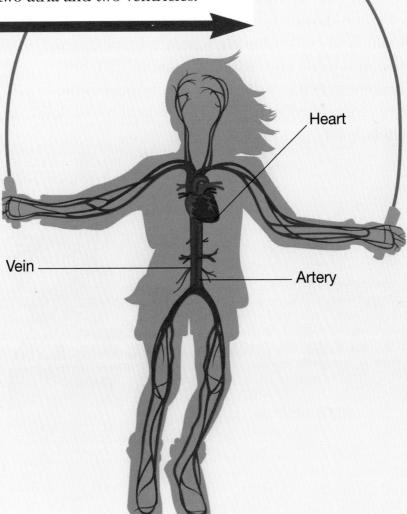

Heart

Vein

Artery

The pumping action of your heart moves blood throughout the body. The right atrium and ventricle receive blood from all parts of your body. This blood is pumped to your lungs through arteries. An *artery* is a blood vessel that carries blood away from the heart.

In your lungs, blood picks up oxygen from the air you breathe. The left atrium and ventricle receive blood rich in oxygen from your lungs through veins. A *vein* is a blood vessel that carries blood to the heart. This blood is pumped from the heart through arteries to all parts of your body.

As blood moves through your body, an exchange takes place between capillaries and body cells. *Capillaries* (KA·puh·lehr·eez) are small blood vessels that connect arteries to veins. Oxygen moves from the blood in the capillaries into body cells.

Carbon dioxide moves from body cells into the blood. Carbon dioxide is a waste gas made by your cells. It is made after oxygen is used by the body. This blood, rich in carbon dioxide, returns to the right atrium through veins. The cycle of blood flow begins again.

- Get plenty of physical activity to make the heart muscle strong.
- Do not eat too many fatty or oily foods to keep arteries clear.
- Do not use tobacco or breathe second-hand smoke.
- Have a plan to lower stress.

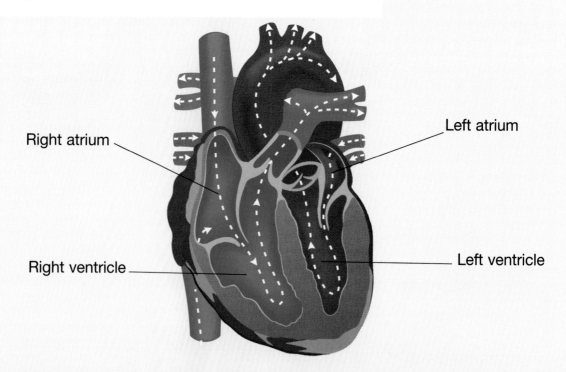

Right atrium

Left atrium

Right ventricle

Left ventricle

How Can I Care for My Respiratory System?

Your **respiratory system** is the body system that helps the body use the air you breathe. When you breathe in, air moves through your mouth or nose. The air moves to your trachea (TRAY·kee·uh) and bronchi. The *bronchi* (BRAHN·ky) are short tubes that carry air from the trachea to both the left and right lung. The bronchi branch into smaller tubes and alveoli. *Alveoli* (al·vee·OH·ly) are small air sacs in the lungs.

The oxygen in the air you breathe moves into capillaries that surround the air sacs. At the same time, carbon dioxide passes from the blood through the walls of capillaries to the air sacs. The carbon dioxide leaves your body when you breathe out.

- Get plenty of physical activity.
- Do not breathe toxic fumes, such as glue.
- Do not use tobacco or breathe secondhand smoke.

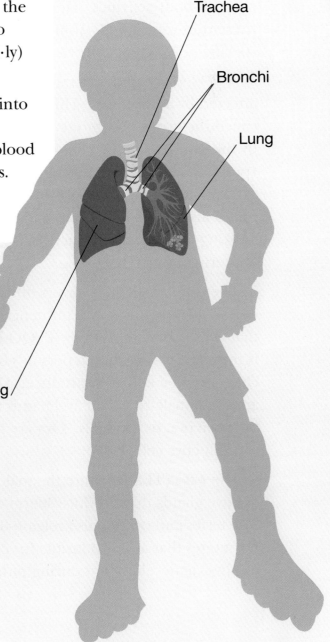

Trachea

Bronchi

Lung

Lung

How Can I Care for My Endocrine System?

The **endocrine** (EN·duh·kruhn) **system** is the body system made up of glands. The glands make special chemicals called hormones. A *hormone* (HOR·mohn) is a chemical that is produced by glands and controls body activities. Hormones are present in your blood. Your glands make specific hormones.

A person's height and rate of growth are affected by a hormone. This hormone is called the growth hormone. It is produced by the pituitary gland. The *pituitary* (puh·TOO·uh·TER·ee) *gland* is an endocrine gland that helps control growth rate. It is found at the base of the brain. You stop growing when your pituitary gland stops delivering growth hormone.

The pituitary gland delivers other hormones. These hormones influence glands that cause puberty. *Puberty* (PYOO·ber·tee) is the stage in life when a person's body changes to be able to reproduce. *Ovaries* are the female reproductive glands that produce ova, or egg cells. Ova are female reproductive cells.

The *testes* (TES·teez) are the male reproductive glands that produce sperm cells. The testes and ovaries also release the hormones that are responsible for changes in physical development during puberty.

- Have regular physical examinations.
- Ask your parents or guardian questions about growth.

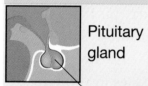

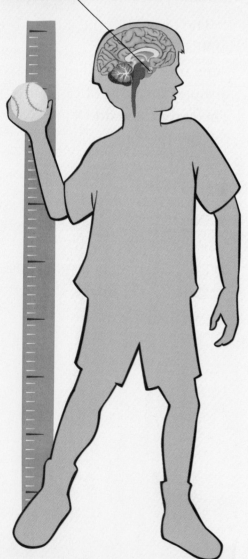

Pituitary gland

Body Systems Crossword Puzzle

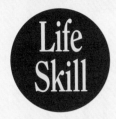

Life Skill

I will care for my body systems.

Materials: Paper, pen or pencil

Directions: Make a cross-word puzzle with at least eight words in it. Use the following vocabulary words and their definitions.

cell	medulla
tissue	spinal cord
organ	atria
body system	ventricles
bone marrow	artery
joint	vein
ligaments	capillaries
tendons	bronchi
voluntary muscles	alveoli
involuntary muscles	hormone
cerebrum	pituitary gland
cerebellum	puberty
	ovaries
	testes

Activity

Lesson 11

Review

Vocabulary

Write a separate sentence using each of the vocabulary words listed on page 72.

Health Content

Write answers to the following:

1. How can you care for your skeletal system? **page 73** For your muscular system? **page 74**
2. How can you care for your nervous system? **page 75** For your digestive system? **page 76**
3. How can you care for your circulatory system? **pages 77–78**
4. How can you care for your respiratory system? **page 79**
5. How can you care for your endocrine system? **page 80**

Steps to Healthful Growth and Aging

Vocabulary

life cycle: the stages of life from birth to death.

mature: to become fully grown or developed.

growth spurt: a rapid increase in height and weight.

critical thinking skills: skills that help you think quickly and decide what to do.

mood swings: changes in emotions caused by hormone levels.

age: to grow older.

death: the loss of life when vital organs no longer work.

grief: discomfort that results from a loss.

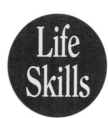

Life Skills

- **I will learn the stages of the life cycle.**
- **I will accept how my body changes as I grow.**
- **I will choose habits for healthful growth and aging.**

Life is a journey. You begin your journey during infancy and pass through different stages until you reach late adulthood. The steps you take along the way determine the quality of life you will have. Right now you are taking steps toward adulthood.

The Lesson Objectives

- Discuss the nine stages in the life cycle.
- Discuss ways you will mature during adolescence.
- List habits to choose now to age in a healthful way.
- Discuss ways to handle grief.

What Are the Stages in the Life Cycle?

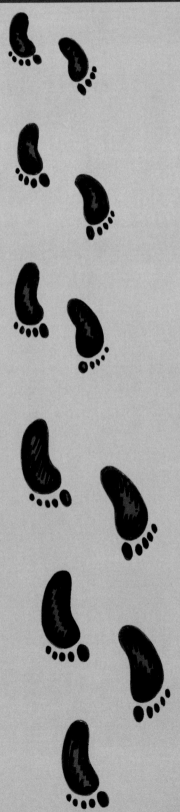

The **life cycle** is the stages of life from birth to death. There are nine stages in the life cycle. In each stage, you grow and learn.

Infancy is the stage of growth from birth to one year. During infancy, you were called an infant. You grew very fast. You might have tripled your birth weight during the first year. You got teeth and they began to break through your gums. You began to notice familiar signs and sounds and enjoyed playing with toys. Your muscles grew. You learned to crawl and you might have begun to walk before your first birthday. You depended on others to meet your needs. In infancy, you learned to trust.

Early childhood is the stage of growth from one to three years. During this stage, you explored your surroundings and adults kept you safe. You became toilet-trained. In early childhood, you learned to show self-control.

Middle childhood is the stage of growth from three to six years. During this stage, you learned that some choices are better than others. You learned which choices to make by watching your parents or guardian. In middle childhood, you learned to tell the difference between right and wrong.

Late childhood is the stage of growth from 6 to 12 years. You are now in this stage of the life cycle. During this stage, you learn many skills. You learn to read, write, and do math. You learn how to help out with household chores. You discover hobbies and special talents to enjoy. In late childhood, you learn to master skills and feel that you can do them well.

Adolescence is the stage of growth from 12 to 18 years. During adolescence, you will have physical, mental, social, and emotional growth. You will have new emotions to understand. Your body will grow and you will work to accept body changes. In adolescence, you learn to accept who you are.

Young adulthood is the stage of growth from 18 to 30 years. Think about people you know who are 18 to 30 years old. They have moved out or will soon move out and live on their own. They spend time in a special relationship. As they get older, they might marry and begin a family. During young adulthood, you will learn how to live on your own and have a lasting relationship.

First adulthood is the stage of growth from 30 to 45 years. Think about people you know in first adulthood. These people might be busy with their jobs. They might be busy raising a family. During first adulthood, you will learn to balance work and family life.

Second adulthood is the stage of growth from 45 to 70 years. Midlife is a term used for this stage. This is because many people have lived about half of their lives when they begin this stage. Think about someone you know who is 45 to 70 years old. People this age look back at the first half of their lives. They were very busy with work and raising a family. Now they have more time to give to their communities. They teach and help others. During second adulthood, you will learn to give back to others.

Late adulthood is the stage of growth from 70 and beyond. Most people who reach late adulthood are healthy. They can participate in activities they enjoy. They enjoy spending time with family. They share memories with their families. They also might talk about death. During late adulthood, people learn to accept death.

When you take the steps of the life cycle you learn:

- To trust.
- To show self-control.
- To tell the difference between right and wrong.
- To master skills and feel capable.
- To accept who you are.
- To support yourself and have a lasting relationship.
- To balance work and family life.
- To give back to others.
- To accept death.

"Picture of Health"

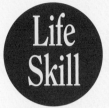

Life Skill

I will choose habits for healthful growth and aging.

Materials: Recent class picture or other picture of yourself, copy of the picture, markers, paper, pen or pencil

Directions: Complete the following activity before you read the next page of this book.

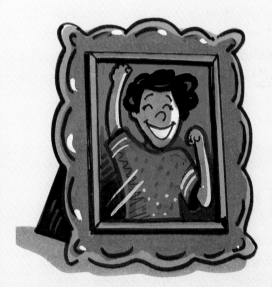

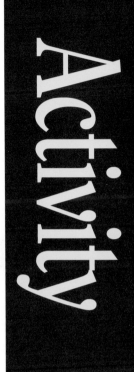

Activity

1. **Study the picture of yourself.** Are you the "picture of health"? Are you physically fit? Do you get plenty of rest and sleep? Do you stay away from cigarette and cigar smoke? Do you practice stress management skills to keep from getting stressed out? Do you eat low-fat foods and cut back on the amount of sugar and salt you eat? Do you use a safety restraint system when riding in a car? Do you relate well with family and friends? Write a paragraph to describe the picture of yourself. Describe your habits and how you look.

2. **Change the picture to show yourself in second adulthood (between the ages of 45 and 70).** Use the markers to change the copy of the picture of yourself. Show what you think you will look like between the ages of 45 and 70. Then write a paragraph that describes what you are like in second adulthood. Talk about your level of wellness. Are you fit? Could you run or walk a mile quickly? Are you underweight? Overweight? About the right weight? Do you relate well to family and friends? Do you breathe easily when you climb stairs?

In What Ways Will I Mature During Adolescence?

Adolescence is the period between late childhood and young adulthood. During adolescence, you will mature in many ways. To **mature** is to become fully grown or developed.

Physical Development

Hormones cause a growth spurt. A **growth spurt** (SPERT) is a rapid increase in height and weight. Girls usually undergo a growth spurt earlier than do boys. Many girls begin their growth spurt about age 11. Some girls do not have their growth spurt until they are 13 or 14. If a girl begins her growth spurt around age 11, she might grow taller than boys her age.

Boys usually do not begin their growth spurt until age 13 or 14 or sometimes older. At this time, boys often grow taller than girls. Their shoulders get wider and their voices become deeper. During adolescence, boys and girls grow at different rates. The rate at which you grow might be very different from the rate at which your friends grow.

Intellectual Development

During adolescence, there is mental growth, too. Your critical thinking skills improve. **Critical thinking skills** are skills that help you think quickly and decide what to do. During adolescence, you will be challenged to use these skills. Your parents or guardian can help you judge the outcomes. As a result, you improve your critical thinking skills. This helps you prepare for early adulthood.

Social Development

During adolescence, you become more interested in your social life. You might be very careful when you choose friends. You are likely to choose friends who have the same interests.

You might feel a strong need to belong. Many adolescents hang out with a group of three or four other adolescents. Being in a group can give you a feeling of security. You can test out your ideas and feelings. But remember not to leave out others. Be open to having friends outside the group. Be open to making friends who are different from you.

Emotional Development

During adolescence, you might have mood swings. **Mood swings** are changes in emotions caused by hormone levels. For example, you might feel relaxed one minute and stressed the next. Or you might suddenly feel like crying or exploding for no reason.

Always choose healthful ways to express emotions. For example, suppose you are angry. Do not explode or hurt others. These actions get you into trouble. Use an I-message to express your emotions to others. Write your feelings in a diary. This helps you express your emotions without harmful outcomes. Part of emotional development is learning to express emotions without harmful outcomes.

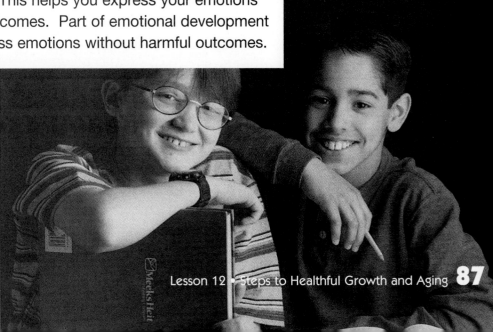

What Habits Can I Choose Now to Age in a Healthful Way?

To **age** is to grow older. Did you know that you are aging right now? You are aging every minute that you are alive. There is something important to know about aging. The habits you choose right now add up as you age. By the time you reach second adulthood, you will see the results of your habits. Remember, second adulthood is the stage of growth from 45 to 70 years. Do you know anyone who is 45 years old? In what condition is this person? What activities does this person enjoy?

What condition do you want to be in when you are 45 years old? Do you want to be able to swim, play golf, shoot baskets, take long walks, or in-line skate? Do you want to be able to climb stairs? To carry boxes and groceries without tiring? Do you want to have a strong heart and clear lungs? Do you want to be at a healthful weight? Do you want to have strong abdominal muscles? If you choose healthful habits now, you can age in a healthful way.

Right now: You get plenty of physical activity.

If you continue this habit into adulthood...

Suppose you get plenty of physical activity right now. You might walk, jog, or run. You might ride your bicycle after school and go in-line skating. You develop the habit of getting plenty of physical activity. Suppose you continue this habit into adulthood. You are less likely to have heart disease. This is because your heart muscle is strong. Your arteries are clear and blood can easily flow through them. You are in good shape. You can participate in and enjoy physical activities.

Life Expectancy

Life expectancy is the number of years a person can expect to live. Most people can expect to live into late adulthood. They can expect to live into their 70s and beyond. This is the length of life that you might expect. But what is the quality of life that you might expect? Your habits influence the quality of life you will have. Your habits right now count.

Right now: You wear sunscreen with a sun protection factor of 15 or more and you stay away from sunlamps and tanning booths.

If you continue these habits into adulthood...

Suppose you enjoy being outdoors. When it is sunny, you wear sunscreen with a sun protection factor (SPF) of 15 or more. You wear a hat and sunglasses. During the hottest part of the day, you stay inside. You say NO if friends suggest a sunlamp or tanning booth. Suppose you continue these habits into adulthood. You are less likely to get skin cancer. You will have fewer wrinkles than your friends who did not use sunscreen. You have smoother skin than your friends who used a sunlamp or tanning booth.

Right now: You do not smoke and you stay away from secondhand smoke.

If you continue these habits into adulthood...

Suppose you never smoke a cigarette. You ask other people not to smoke cigarettes, cigars, or pipes around you. If you eat out, you eat in restaurants where smoking is not allowed. Suppose you continue these habits into second adulthood. Your teeth will be white and your gums will stay healthy. You will have fewer wrinkles than your friends who smoked. You do not cough. You are less likely to have heart disease and lung cancer.

Right now: You eat plenty of grains, fruits, and vegetables.

If you continue this habit into adulthood...

Suppose you eat whole wheat cereal, granola, or oatmeal for breakfast. You eat a bran muffin, too. You have several servings of fruits and vegetables throughout the day. You have other servings from the grain group. This helps you have a daily bowel movement. Suppose you continue this habit into adulthood. You are less likely to have problems with digestion. You are less likely to have colon cancer.

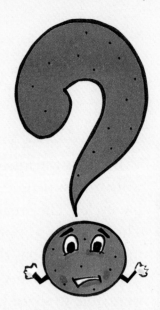

Did You Know....?

Smoking contributes to more than 30 percent of all cancer deaths. Cancer is a leading cause of death.

Protect your health. Do not begin the habit of smoking. Do not smoke even one cigarette. If you have ever tried smoking, pledge that you will not smoke again.

Smoking right now is risky.

How Can I Handle Grief?

Death is the loss of life when vital organs no longer work. Most people live through the nine stages in the life cycle. They reach late adulthood and then die. Their organs stop working. Perhaps an older person in your family has died. Your family might have had time to prepare for this person's death. Perhaps you were able to share your feelings with this person. This person might have shared feelings with you.

When someone dies, you have grief. **Grief** (GREEF) is discomfort that results from a loss. When you feel grief, you have many emotions. You might have disbelief or anger. You might feel very sad and cry. When you feel grief, there can be body changes. You might have headaches or a hard time sleeping. You might have a hard time doing schoolwork.

Ways to Handle Grief

- Express your emotions in a healthful way. Write about how you are feeling. Talk with your parents, guardian, or another adult. Spend time with friends who will listen.

- Choose behaviors to keep your body healthy. Get plenty of physical activity. Get plenty of rest and sleep. Eat healthful foods.

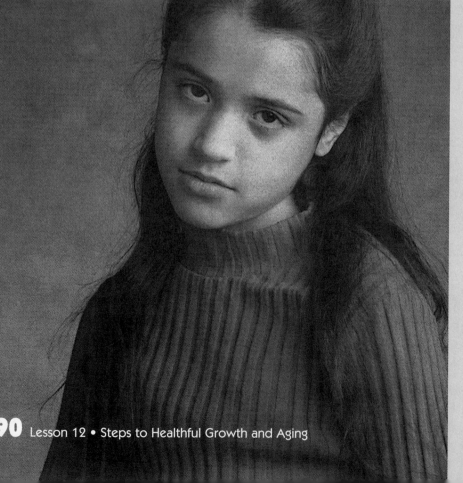

Use... Guidelines for Making Responsible Decisions™

A classmate has a sunlamp. Your classmate says you will look sharp with a tan. You mention the health risks that go along with using a sunlamp. Your classmate says, "You don't have to worry about skin cancer until you're older."

Use a separate sheet of paper. Answer "yes" or "no" to each of the following questions. Explain each answer.

1. Is it healthful for you to use a sunlamp?
2. Is it safe for you to use a sunlamp?
3. Do you follow rules and laws if you use a sunlamp?
4. Do you show respect for yourself and others if you use a sunlamp?
5. Do you follow your family's guidelines if you use a sunlamp?
6. Do you show good character if you use a sunlamp?

What is the responsible decision to make?

Lesson 12

Review

Vocabulary

Write a separate sentence using each of the vocabulary words listed on page 82.

Health Content

Write answers to the following:

1. What are the nine stages in the life cycle? **pages 83–84**
2. In what ways will you mature during adolescence? **pages 86–87**
3. Why do adolescents sometimes have mood swings? **page 87**
4. What are four habits you can choose now to help you age in a healthful way? **pages 88–89**
5. How can you handle your grief when someone dies? **page 90**

Discover Your Learning Style

Vocabulary

unique: one of a kind.

learning style: the way you gain skills and information.

Braille system: a way of touch reading and writing used by a person who is blind.

sign language: a way of communicating in which the fingers and hands are used to form letters and words.

learning disability: a disorder that causes someone to have difficulty learning.

tutor: a person who gives individual help to a student.

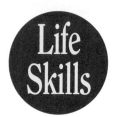

Life Skills

- **I will be glad that I am unique.**
- **I will discover my learning style.**

To be **unique** (yoo·NEEK) is to be one of a kind. You are unique because no one is just like you. That is why it is best not to compare yourself to others. Instead, you should try to be the very best person you can be. You do this by always trying your best.

The Lesson Objectives

- Explain why you are unique.
- Discuss ways to help you learn.
- Explain how to use the Braille system and sign language.
- Tell the kinds of support that might be needed by someone who has a learning disability.

Why Am I Unique?

You received some traits from your biological mother. You received some traits from your biological father. Your heredity is the sum of these traits. No one else has the same sum of traits. Suppose you have a brother or sister who has the same biological mother and father as you. Your brother or sister received traits, too. But the sum of these traits is different. Your brother or sister might have some of the same traits as you. But some of his or her traits will be different. Your personalities might be alike in some ways. Your experiences and interests might be alike. But in other ways they are different. Your brother or sister does not have the same private thoughts as you do.

Suppose you have an identical twin. An identical twin does have the same heredity as you. But an identical twin still will be different. Identical twins are not born at exactly the same time. They do not have exactly the same experiences. For this reason, they often have different personalities. Even if they look very much alike you can tell them apart. They often develop different interests. Their private thoughts are not the same.

Be glad that you are unique. Try to be the best you can be. Then other people benefit from knowing you. They will never meet someone who is just like you. They can enjoy ways in which you are different from them. Be glad that other people are unique. Try to learn what is unique about each person. Encourage others to be at their best.

You Are Unique Because...

No one adds up

- **+ inherited traits**
- **+ personality**
- **+ experiences**
- **+ interests**
- **+ private thoughts**

the way YOU do.

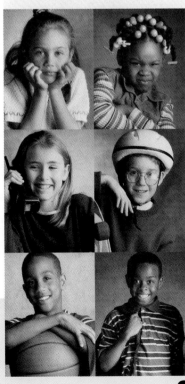

What Are Ways to Help Me Learn?

Your **learning style** is the way you gain skills and information. You learn by reading, listening, and getting involved. Here are ways to help you learn.

Learn by reading. Do you spend much time reading? Reading is one of the best ways to get skills and information. This is why you should read often.

- Try to remember key points when you read.
- Take notes on what you have read.
- Study the pictures or diagrams that go with the words.
- Look up the definitions of words you do not know.
- Discuss what you read with your parents or guardian.

Learn by listening. Do you understand and remember what you hear? You can learn from conversations. You can learn from words that you hear in movies. You can learn from listening to music and different sounds.

- Pay careful attention to what you hear.
- Sit or stand close enough to hear.
- Listen with your eyes as well as your ears.
- Ask questions if you do not understand.

Learn by doing. Do you enjoy being an active learner? Learning by doing is one of the best ways to learn.

- Pay close attention to the directions.
- Watch a mentor and copy what the mentor does.
- Practice doing the same skill more than once.

Using Braille

The **Braille** (BRAYL) **system** is a way of touch reading and writing used by a person who is blind. Raised dots stand for letters of the alphabet and are grouped together to form words. A person who uses the Braille system touches these dots to identify the letters.

Using Sign Language

Sign language is a way of communicating in which the fingers and hands are used to form letters and words. People who are hearing impaired and those with whom they speak might use this way to communicate. They must know the sign language alphabet.

The Sign Language Alphabet

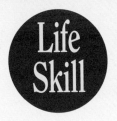

Life Skill

I will discover my learning style.

Materials: None

Directions: The Sign Language Alphabet appears below. Practice signing one of the life skills that appears on page 8 or 9. Then sign for the class. Classmates can guess which life skill you signed.

Activity

The Sign Language Alphabet

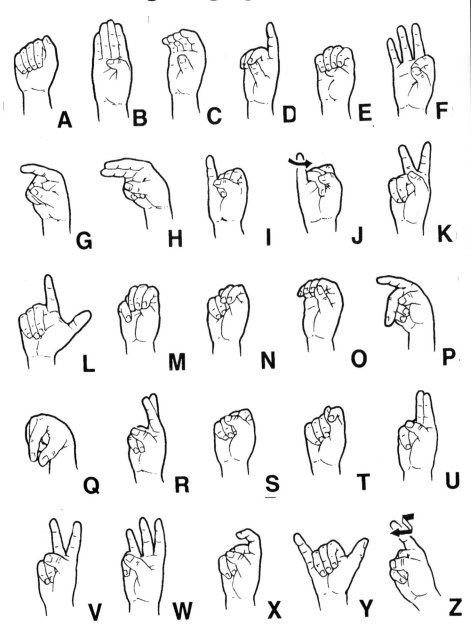

What Kinds of Support Are Needed by Someone with a Learning Disability?

A **learning disability** is a disorder that causes someone to have difficulty learning. Do you have a learning disability? Do you have classmates who have learning disabilities?

There are different kinds of learning disabilities. Some young people who have learning disabilities do not understand what they read. They might see letters upside down. They might change the order of letters and numbers. Other young people who have learning disabilities might have difficulty putting things in correct order.

Other young people who have learning disabilities are very restless. They cannot sit still for very long. They have a short attention span.

Young people who have learning disabilities need support to learn. They might take classes in a learning center at school. There are fewer students in the class. They get extra help from the teachers in the learning center. Some young people who have learning disabilities have a tutor. A **tutor** is a person who gives individual help to a student.

Young people who have learning disabilities need social support, too. They need to be accepted by their peers. They need to feel like they belong. For example, suppose a group project is given by the teacher. They need to feel wanted by the other students in the group. They need to do a part of the project.

Young people who have learning disabilities need emotional support. They might want to give up. Other students can encourage them to keep trying.

What Is Cooperative Learning?

During the school day, you might join in on cooperative learning. Cooperative learning is working together with classmates on something. You might work with your classmates on a project. The classmates with whom you work might have different skills. You work as a team. You decide who will do what based on the skills of those with whom you work. Cooperative learning gives you a chance to practice social skills. You practice teamwork, too.

No One Adds Up Like I Do

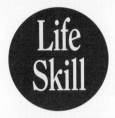

Life Skill

I will be glad that I am unique.

Materials: Poster board or large sheet of paper, markers

Directions: Review the equation in the margin on page 93. The equation shows why you are unique.

1. **Create an equation to show why you add up to be unique.**
2. **Write your equation on poster board or a large sheet of paper. Include:**
   - One of your inherited traits
   - One of your personality traits
   - One unusual experience you have had
   - One of your special interests
   - One of your private thoughts (choose one you want to share)
3. **Share your equation with your classmates.** What parts of your equation were like those of classmates? What parts of your equation were different from those of classmates?

Activity

Lesson 13

Review

Vocabulary

Write a separate sentence using each of the vocabulary words listed on page 92.

Health Content

Write answers to the following:

1. Why are you unique? **page 93**
2. What are ways to help you learn when you read? When you listen? When you get involved? **page 94**
3. How do you use the Braille system? **page 94**
4. How do you use sign language? **page 94**
5. What kinds of support might be needed by someone who has a learning disability? **page 96**

Unit 3 Review

Health Content

Review your answers for each Lesson Review in this unit. Write answers to the following questions.

1. At what age do your bones stop growing? **Lesson 11 page 73**

2. Why do you need to eat foods that contain fiber? **Lesson 11 page 76**

3. What are the bronchi? **Lesson 11 page 79**

4. At what ages will you be in adolescence? **Lesson 12 page 84**

5. When do boys begin their growth spurt? **Lesson 12 page 86**

6. What causes mood swings? **Lesson 12 page 87**

7. What can you do to handle grief? **Lesson 12 page 90**

8. How might a person who is hearing impaired talk to someone? **Lesson 13 page 94**

9. How might a person who is blind read a book? **Lesson 13 page 94**

10. How might you show support to a classmate who has a learning disability? **Lesson 13 page 96**

Guidelines for Making Responsible Decisions™

You have a school project that you are working on with a classmate. You are gluing pictures from a magazine on poster board. Your friend likes the strong smell of glue. But you are worried about the fumes. You open the window to get fresh air. Use a separate sheet of paper. Answer "yes" or "no" to each of the following questions. Explain each answer.

1. Is it healthful for you to open the window to get fresh air?

2. Is it safe for you to open the window to get fresh air?

3. Do you follow rules and laws if you open the window to get fresh air?

4. Do you show respect for yourself and others if you open the window to get fresh air?

5. Do you follow your family's guidelines if you open the window to get fresh air?

6. Do you show good character if you open the window to get fresh air?

What is the responsible decision to make?

Family Involvement

With your parents or guardian, make a list of five study habits on which you can work.

Vocabulary

Number a sheet of paper from 1–10. Read each definition. Next to each number on your sheet of paper, write the vocabulary word that matches the definition.

endocrine system	age
life cycle	unique
critical thinking skills	circulatory system
Braille system	sign language
learning disability	growth spurt

1. The body system that transports oxygen, food, and waste through the body. **Lesson 11**
2. The stages of life from birth to death. **Lesson 12**
3. To grow older. **Lesson 12**
4. Skills that help you think quickly and decide what to do. **Lesson 12**
5. A way of touch reading and writing used by a person who is blind. **Lesson 13**
6. The body system made up of glands. **Lesson 11**
7. A disorder that causes someone to have difficulty learning. **Lesson 13**
8. One of a kind. **Lesson 13**
9. A rapid increase in height and weight. **Lesson 12**
10. A way of communicating in which fingers and hands are used to form letters and words. **Lesson 13**

Health Literacy

Effective Communication

Make a sympathy card that might be sent to someone who is grieving the death of a family member.

Self-Directed Learning

Visit your local library. Check to see what books on tape the library has. Select a book on tape and listen to it.

Critical Thinking

Explain why a person who is not hearing impaired might learn sign language.

Responsible Citizenship

Get permission from your parents or guardian. Offer to tutor a younger brother or sister or a child in a lower grade level than you.

Multicultural Health

In some cultures, growing up is cause for a celebration. For example, in our culture we celebrate growing up with birthday celebrations. Research another culture to find out how it celebrates growing up. Write a paragraph about it.

Unit 4

Nutrition

Follow Those Guidelines

Vocabulary

nutrients: substances in food that your body uses for energy and for growth and repair of cells.

food group: foods that contain the same nutrients.

Food Guide Pyramid: a guide that shows how many servings are needed from each food group each day.

balanced diet: a daily diet that includes the correct number of servings from the food groups in the Food Guide Pyramid.

Dietary Guidelines: suggested goals for eating to help you stay healthy and live longer.

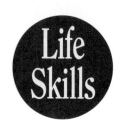

Life Skills

- **I will eat the correct number of servings from the Food Guide Pyramid.**
- **I will follow the Dietary Guidelines.**
- **I will read food labels.**

Your diet is made up of the foods you eat and the beverages you drink. To have high level wellness, you need to have six kinds of nutrients in your diet. You also need to follow guidelines when choosing foods and beverages. Knowing how to read food labels helps you follow guidelines.

The Lesson Objectives

- Name foods that are sources of the six kinds of nutrients.
- Name the number of servings you need every day from each food group in the Food Guide Pyramid.
- Name tips that help you follow the Dietary Guidelines.
- Explain how to use a food label to find facts you need to follow the Dietary Guidelines.

What Foods Are Sources of the Six Kinds of Nutrients?

Nutrients are substances in food that your body uses for energy and for growth and repair of cells. You need to eat foods that are sources of the six kinds of nutrients.

Kinds of Nutrients

Nutrients	Food Sources
Proteins are nutrients your body uses for growth and repair of cells and to supply energy.	Eggs, cheese, milk, fish, beans, nuts, turkey, chicken, beef, pork
Carbohydrates are nutrients that are the most useful supply of energy for your body.	Bread, rice, potatoes, cereals, noodles, fruits, vegetables
Fats are nutrients your body uses for energy and to help store some vitamins.	Hamburger, steak, pork, margarine, butter, milk, ice cream, peanut butter, salad dressing
Vitamins are nutrients that help regulate body processes and fight disease. They help promote the growth of new cells.	Fruits and vegetables, milk, meat, breads, cereals, eggs, vitamin supplements
Minerals are nutrients that help regulate body processes and build new cells. Fluoride is a mineral that is added to drinking water to make teeth strong.	Fruits and vegetables, milk, meat, breads, cereals, eggs, mineral supplements
Water is a nutrient that helps with digestion, makes up most of your blood, helps remove waste products, and helps regulate body temperature.	Drinking water, milk, soups, juices, fruits, vegetables

How Many Servings Do I Need Every Day from Each Food Group in the Food Guide Pyramid?

A **food group** is foods that contain the same nutrients. The **Food Guide Pyramid** is a guide that shows how many servings are needed from each food group each day. A **balanced diet** is a daily diet that includes the correct number of servings from the food groups in the Food Guide Pyramid.

The Milk, Yogurt, and Cheese Group
(2–3 servings)

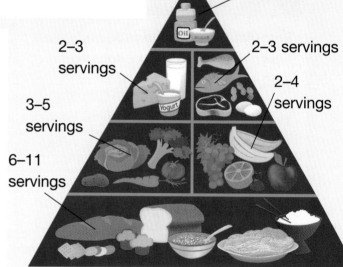

This food group is a source of calcium and phosphorous (FAHS· for·uhs). These two minerals make teeth and bones strong. Vitamin D often is added to milk to help your body use calcium.

Fats, Oils, and Sweets
Use sparingly

2–3 servings

2–3 servings

2–4 servings

3–5 servings

6–11 servings

The Meat, Poultry, Fish, Dry Beans, Eggs, and Nuts Group
(2–3 servings of two or three ounces)

Beef, pork, fish, and poultry are in this food group. Beans, eggs, and nuts also are in this food group. Foods in this food group are sources of protein, vitamins, and minerals. They contain B vitamins for growth. Iron is a mineral provided by this food group.

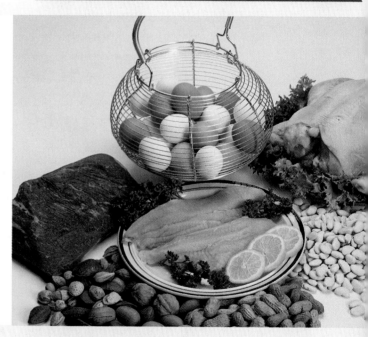

The Vegetable Group
(3–5 servings)

Vegetables supply vitamins, minerals, and carbohydrates (kar·boh·HY·drayts). Deep orange and dark green vegetables provide vitamin A. Vitamin A helps keep your eyes and skin healthy. It also helps with night vision. Vegetables are a good source of fiber. Fiber is the part of grains and plant foods that cannot be digested. Fiber helps move waste through your body. Eating foods with fiber each day can help you have a daily bowel movement.

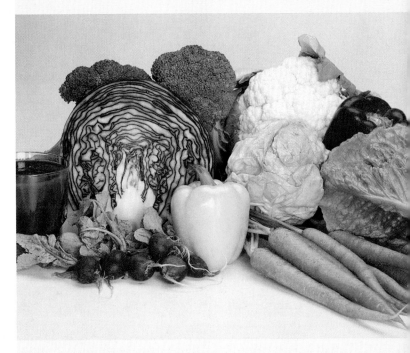

The Fruit Group
(2–4 servings)

Fruits also supply vitamins, minerals, and carbohydrates. Grapefruit, oranges, lemons, limes, and tomatoes provide vitamin C. Vitamin C helps you have healthy gums and blood vessels. Fruits also are good sources of fiber.

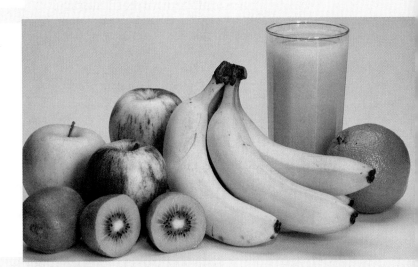

The Bread, Cereal, Rice, and Pasta Group
(6–11 servings)

This food group contains grains. Grains are seeds from certain plants. Examples of grains are wheat, oats, barley, rye, rice, and corn. Foods made from grains are breads, pastas, and cereal. They are a good source of carbohydrates, vitamins, and minerals. They also are a good source of fiber.

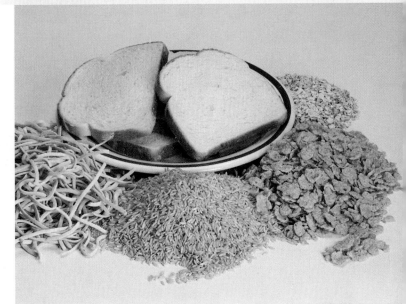

What Are Tips I Can Use to Follow the Dietary Guidelines?

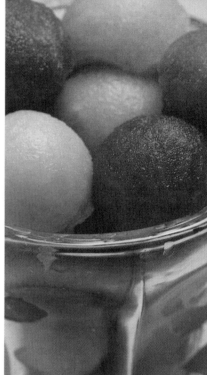

The seven **Dietary Guidelines** are suggested goals for eating to help you stay healthy and live longer.

Goal 1: Eat a variety of foods.

Goal 2: Balance the food you eat with physical activity—stay at a healthful weight.

Goal 3: Eat few fatty foods.

Goal 4: Eat plenty of grains, vegetables, and fruits.

Goal 5: Eat small amounts of sugar.

Goal 6: Use little salt.

Goal 7: Do not drink alcohol.

Eat Fewer Fatty Foods

Goal 3 concerns fatty foods. There are two kinds of fats in foods. *Saturated* (SA·chuh·RAYT·uhd) *fats* are fats in foods that come from animals. These fats are found in foods like steak, hamburger, liver, and ham. Dairy products such as whole milk, cream, butter, cheese, and ice cream contain these fats. *Unsaturated fats* are fats in foods that come from vegetables, nuts, seeds, poultry, and fish. Corn oil and peanut oil contain this kind of fat.

Limit the amount of fats in your diet. Fats can stick to artery walls and cause heart disease. Fats are high in calories. They cause weight gain. Staying at a healthful weight lowers the risk of cancer.

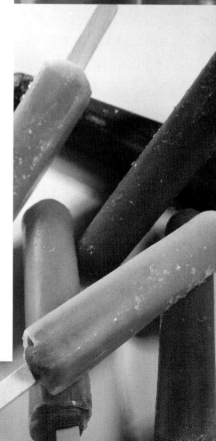

- Eat small portions of meat and pork.
- Cut off the fat from meat and pork before cooking.
- Eat foods that are baked or broiled rather than fried.
- Choose low-fat dairy products, such as low-fat yogurt.

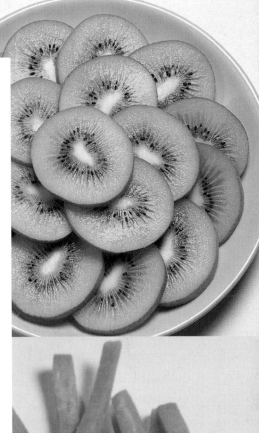

Eat Plenty of Grains, Vegetables, and Fruits

Grains are complex carbohydrates. *Complex carbohydrates* are nutrients that provide long-lasting energy. Grains are rich in B vitamins and in minerals. Grains contain fiber to help you have a daily bowel movement. This helps reduce the risk of cancer.

Vegetables and fruits are sources of vitamins, minerals, and fibers. Broccoli contains substances that reduce the risk of some cancers. Citrus fruits contain vitamin C. Vitamin C helps your body resist disease. Vegetables and fruits are low in calories. They help you stay at a healthful weight.

- Eat cereal for breakfast and for snacks.
- Eat granola bars instead of candy bars.
- Drink fruit and vegetable juice instead of soda.
- Eat fruits for snacks and desserts.

Eat Small Amounts of Sugar

Foods that contain lots of sugar are high in calories. If you pig out on them, you get full. You might not eat foods that provide vitamins and minerals. You might gain weight. Foods that contain sugar increase the chance of having cavities.

- Do not add sugar to food.
- Choose cereal that is not sugar-coated.

Use Little Salt

You do not need much salt. There is already salt in canned foods.

- Do not add salt to foods.
- Buy foods that are labeled "reduced salt."
- Stay away from foods on which you see chunks of salt, such as salted pretzels.

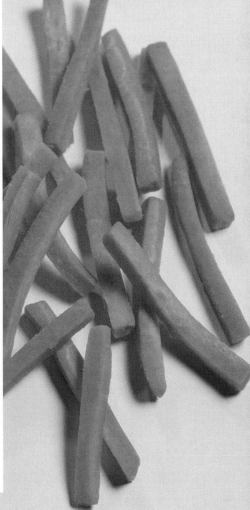

What Facts on a Food Label Can I Use to Follow the Dietary Guidelines?

A *food label* is a list of facts on a food container required by federal law. The law requires that a food label state the name of the food and the amount of the food in the package. The name, address, and zip code of the company that makes and packages the food must be listed. The *ingredients* (in·GREE·dee·uhnts) *listing* is the list of ingredients that are in the food or beverage. The ingredient that appears first makes up the largest amount of the food. *Nutrition Facts* is a panel on a food label that gives facts about the food or beverage.

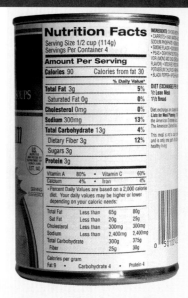

Facts on a Food Label That Help You Follow the Dietary Guidelines

The ingredients listing tells you if the food or beverage has:

- **Grains** (Goal 4: Eat plenty of grains, vegetables, and fruits.)
- **Sugar** (Goal 5: Eat small amounts of sugar.)
- **Salt or sodium** (Goal 6: Use little salt.)

The Nutrition Facts panel tells you:

- **How many calories are in a serving** (Goal 2: Balance the food you eat with physical activity—stay at a healthful weight.)
- **How much fat is in a serving** (Goal 3: Eat few fatty foods.)
- **How much salt is in a serving** (Goal 6: Use little salt.)
- **How much carbohydrate is in a serving** (Goal 1: Eat a variety of foods.)
- **How much protein is in a serving** (Goal 1: Eat a variety of foods.)
- **How much vitamin A and vitamin C are in a serving** (Goal 1: Eat a variety of foods.)
- **How much calcium and iron are in a serving** (Goal 1: Eat a variety of foods.)

Read a Food Label

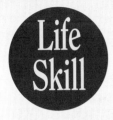

Life Skill

I will read food labels.

Materials: A food label, ingredients listing, poster board, markers

Directions: Follow the steps to learn how reading food labels helps you follow the Dietary Guidelines.

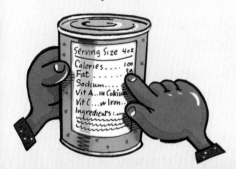

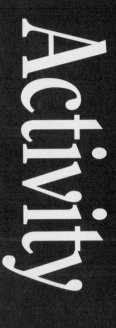

Activity

1. **Get a food label from the container of a food or beverage.** Be sure you have the ingredients listing and the Nutrition Facts panel.

2. **Tape the ingredients listing and the Nutrition Facts panel to the middle of a piece of poster board.**

3. **Write the seven Dietary Guidelines on the side of the poster board.**

4. **Draw an arrow from each guideline to a part of the food label.** The arrow should point to facts that help you decide if the food or beverage is healthful. For example, Goal 3 is "Eat few fatty foods." Draw an arrow from this goal to the place on the Nutrition Facts panel that reads, "Calories from Fat."

Lesson 14

Review

Vocabulary

Write a separate sentence using each of the vocabulary words listed on page 102.

Health Content

Write answers to the following:

1. What foods are sources of protein? Of carbohydrates? Of fats? Of vitamins? Of minerals? Of water? **page 103**

2. How many servings do you need each day from each food group in the Food Guide Pyramid? **pages 104–105**

3. What are tips to help you eat fewer fats? To eat plenty of grains, vegetables, and fruits? **page 106**

4. What are tips to help you eat small amounts of sugar? To use less salt? **page 107**

5. What facts on a food label can help you follow the Dietary Guidelines? **page 108**

Food Choices Count

Vocabulary

ethnic food: a food eaten by people of a specific culture.

fast food restaurant: a place that serves food quickly.

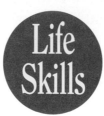

Life Skills

- I will eat healthful meals and snacks.
- I will choose healthful foods if I eat at fast food restaurants.

Suppose you are choosing between a hamburger and a chicken burrito for lunch. How would you choose? Suppose you are choosing between a candy bar and an apple for a snack. How would you choose? All your food choices count. Your food choices must add up to a balanced diet.

The Lesson Objectives

- Discuss factors that influence your food choices.
- Outline steps to follow to plan meals and snacks for one day.
- Name guidelines to use when you order foods at a fast food restaurant.

What Factors Influence Your Food Choices?

On a separate sheet of paper, make a list of the foods you ate yesterday. Why did you choose certain foods? Five factors influence your food choices.

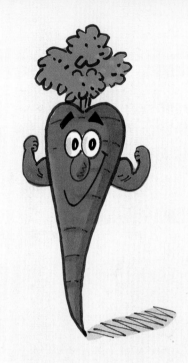

Your Personal Likes You choose certain foods because you like their smell, taste, and texture. For example, you might enjoy the smell of pizza. You might enjoy the texture of mashed potatoes. Foods that are barbecued might taste good to you. As a result, you choose these foods more often than others.

Your Commitment to Health Suppose you want to be healthy. You might eat unsalted popcorn instead of popcorn with salt. You might eat cereal that is not coated with sugar. You might drink fruit juices instead of soft drinks. If you are not committed to health, it can show in your food choices.

Where You Live Certain foods are grown in different areas because of the type of soil and climate. If you live in Florida, you might drink fresh orange juice. If you live in parts of Texas, you might eat more beef because the land is used to raise cattle. If you live near a large body of water, you might eat more fish. When you travel to another area, you might want to try new foods.

What Foods Are in Season Many foods are easier and cheaper to buy when they are in season. For example, strawberries and corn are grown at certain times of the year.

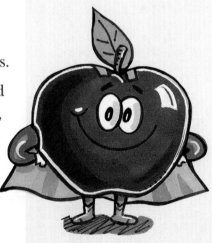

Your Family's Eating Habits Your family might have favorite dishes. Perhaps some of these dishes were prepared by your grandparents. Your family might enjoy ethnic foods. An **ethnic food** is a food eaten by people of a specific culture.

How Do I Plan Meals and Snacks for One Day?

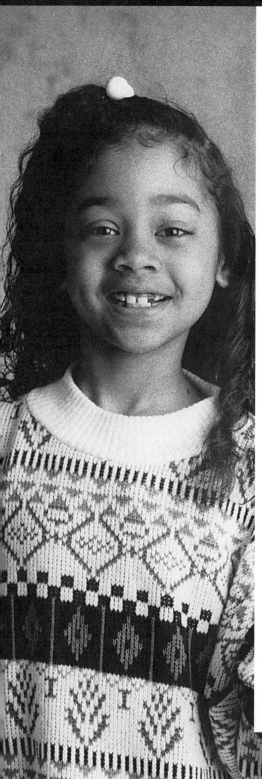

These are the steps to follow to plan meals and snacks for one day.

Plan the number of meals and snacks you will have.
You might eat breakfast, lunch, and dinner with snacks between. You might eat five smaller meals and no snacks. Think about what time you will eat.

Use the Food Guide Pyramid to choose foods and beverages for the meals and snacks you have planned.

Make certain you get the number of servings you need from each food group.

- 2–3 servings from the Milk, Yogurt, and Cheese Group
- 2–3 servings of two or three ounces each from the Meat, Poultry, Fish, Dry Beans, Eggs, and Nut Group
- 3–5 servings from the Vegetable Group
- 2–4 servings from the Fruit Group
- 6–11 servings from the Bread, Cereal, Rice, and Pasta Group

Use the Dietary Guidelines to check out your food and beverage choices.

Goal 1: Eat a variety of foods.

Goal 2: Balance the food you eat with physical activity—stay at a healthful weight.

Goal 3: Eat few fatty foods.

Goal 4: Eat plenty of grains, vegetables, and fruits.

Goal 5: Eat small amounts of sugar.

Goal 6: Use little salt.

Goal 7: Do not drink alcohol.

Make changes if you have chosen foods and beverages that do not follow the Dietary Guidelines.
Suppose you had a doughnut and hot chocolate for breakfast. The doughnut is high in fats and sugar. It is not rich in vitamins and minerals. The hot chocolate was made with milk. Milk has calcium in it. It counts as a serving from the dairy group. But do not eat the doughnut. Eat cereal that is not coated with sugar. Choose one that has plenty of grains. Or eat healthful leftovers. Tuna casserole has protein and carbohydrates. Have some fruit for breakfast.

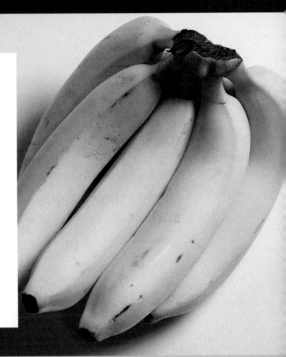

Snack Attack

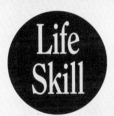

Life Skill I will eat healthful meals and snacks.

Materials: None
Directions: Complete this activity to learn ideas for healthful snacks.

Activity

1. **You and your classmates will stand.**
2. **One classmate begins by saying, "I am having a snack attack and I am going to eat..."** This classmate will name a healthful snack.
3. **The second classmate will say, "I am having a snack attack and I am going to eat...(what the first classmate said) or... (The second classmate names another healthful snack)."**
4. **Continue.** A classmate must sit down if he or she cannot name the snacks the other classmates named. The snacks must be named in the correct order.

What Are Guidelines to Use When I Order Foods at Fast Food Restaurants?

A **fast food restaurant** is a place that serves food quickly. Many fast food restaurants have a drive-through window. You can order, pay, and get your foods and beverages without going inside the restaurant. Some fast food restaurants deliver. Use these guidelines to order foods and beverages at fast food restaurants.

- **Order foods and beverages that contain vitamins and minerals.** Order a baked potato. A baked potato is a good source of potassium. Order skim milk or low-fat milk instead of soda pop. Milk is a good source of calcium and vitamin D.

- **Ask to have salt and butter left off your order.** Suppose you get popcorn at a movie theatre. Order it with no butter. Do not add salt.

- **Do not order more than one fatty food in a meal.** Sometimes you might crave a fatty food. It is OK to eat fatty foods now and then. But do not order several fatty foods at one time. If you order a hamburger, skip the French fries. If you order chili with meat, skip the melted cheese on top.

- **Blot off extra fat from your order.** Suppose you get pizza. Blot it with a napkin. This takes off some of the extra fat. Suppose you order French fries. Put them on a napkin. The napkin might absorb some of the oils in which they were cooked.

- **Order something green.** Order a vegetable. You might get a salad or a side of broccoli.

- **Order foods that are cooked in a healthful way.** Suppose you go to a fast food restaurant that serves chicken. Order it roasted or broiled instead of fried.

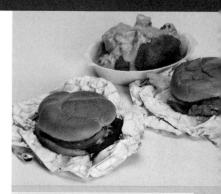

If you order a hamburger, skip the French fries.

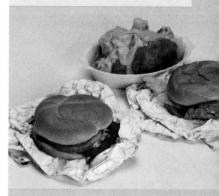

A baked potato is a good source of potassium.

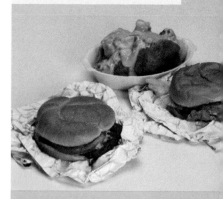

Pass the French Fries

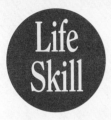

Life Skill

I will choose healthful foods if I eat at fast food restaurants.

Materials: Container of French fries, napkins

Directions: Complete the following activity to learn why you should limit the number of fried foods you order.

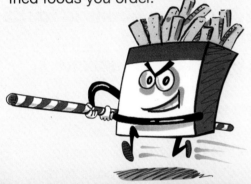

Activity

1. **Several classmates can volunteer to hold French fries in their hands.** They should close the hand in which the French fries were held. Then they can put the French fries back in the container.

2. **Ask the classmates who were holding the French fries in their hands to shake the hand of a classmate.**

3. **Ask those classmates who participated to tell how their hands feel.** Most likely, they will say "sticky." Potatoes are not sticky, but frying potatoes in oil makes them sticky. Fried foods can stick to artery walls.

4. **Name five fried foods that are served at fast food restaurants.**

Lesson 15

Review

Vocabulary

Write a separate sentence using each of the vocabulary words listed on page 110.

Health Content

Write answers to the following:

1. What are five factors that influence your food choices? **page 111**

2. What are steps you can follow to plan meals and snacks for one day? **pages 112–113**

3. What are six guidelines you can use when you order foods and beverages at fast food restaurants? **page 114**

4. How can you get rid of the extra oil if you order fried foods? **page 114**

5. Why should you limit the number of fried foods you order? **page 115**

Be a Food and Beverage Detective

Vocabulary

foodborne illness: an illness caused by eating foods or drinking beverages that contain germs.

table manners: polite ways to eat.

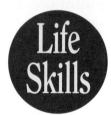

Life Skills

- **I will protect myself and others from germs in foods and beverages.**
- **I will use table manners.**

There are two ways you can become ill from eating foods or drinking beverages. First, you can eat or drink foods and beverages that are spoiled or not cooked enough. Second, you can eat foods or drink beverages that contain germs from other people. There are ways to keep from getting germs when eating foods or drinking beverages.

The Lesson Objectives

- Discuss ways to prevent foodborne illnesses.
- Tell ways to keep from spreading your germs when you share foods and beverages.
- Name good table manners you should practice.

What Are Ways to Prevent Foodborne Illnesses?

A **foodborne illness** is an illness caused by eating foods or drinking beverages that contain germs. Symptoms include diarrhea, nausea, vomiting, and cramps. Treatment includes drinking water and other liquids, and getting bed rest.

Do Not Eat Foods and Drink Beverages That Are Spoiled

- Do not eat foods and drink beverages that smell bad.
- Do not eat foods and drink beverages that are discolored.
- Do not eat foods that are bruised.
- Do not eat foods and drink beverages in containers that are dented, leaking, or bulging.
- Do not eat foods and drink beverages that are sold after the expiration date that is on the container.

Prepare Foods in a Safe Way

- Wash your hands before you handle food.
- Scrub your cutting board after each use.
- Wash fruits and vegetables before you eat them or make juice.
- Cook meat thoroughly.
- Do not let juices from uncooked chicken get on other foods.
- Do not eat foods or drink beverages that have been thawed and refrozen.

Store Foods in a Safe Way

- Put frozen foods you have just bought in the refrigerator right away.
- Set your refrigerator at 40°F or lower.
- Thaw frozen food in your refrigerator and not on your counter.
- Put leftovers in your refrigerator within an hour and a half after they are served.

How Can I Keep from Spreading Germs When I Share Foods and Beverages?

Do you eat lunch with friends? Do you have a snack after school with friends? There are ways to share foods and beverages without spreading germs.

Wash your hands with soap and water before preparing or sharing food. Your fingers and hands touch many objects throughout the day. You might cover your mouth when you cough or cover your nose if you sneeze. You might shake the hand of someone who has germs on his or her hand.

Do not cough or sneeze on foods or beverages. Turn your head if you are going to cough or sneeze. Use a tissue. Wash your hands with soap and water after a cough or sneeze.

Do not use your fingers to taste food you are making. Suppose you are making pudding. Germs can get into the mixture if you use your fingers to taste it.

Do not use a spoon or fork more than once to taste food you are making. Suppose you are making chili. You use a spoon and taste the chili to see if it has enough chili powder in it. You add more chili powder. Then you use the same spoon to taste it again. Germs from your mouth get into the chili.

Share food by cutting off a bite or portion from a part of food you did not eat. Then germs from your mouth do not get on the food you give someone else.

Share beverages by pouring them into separate glasses before you give them to someone else. Do not take a drink from soda pop and then give the can to someone else. Germs from your mouth are on the can.

Canker Sores and Fever Blisters

Suppose someone has canker (KANG-ker) sores in his or her mouth or fever blisters on his or her lips. These can be caused by one of the herpes viruses. Now suppose this person drinks from a can of soda pop. Then this person offers you a drink from the same can. If you drink from the same can, germs from this person's mouth and lips get into your body.

Dip Tip

Suppose you are snacking with friends. There is a bowl of tortillas and a bowl of dip. Use a spoon and place dip on your plate. Dip the tortillas in the dip on your plate.

What Are Good Table Manners I Should Practice?

Table manners are polite ways to eat. Having good table manners helps you look polished. Other people see that you are polite and that you know what to do around other people. When you have good table manners, you keep your self-respect. You feel good about the way you behave around others. Practice the following table manners.

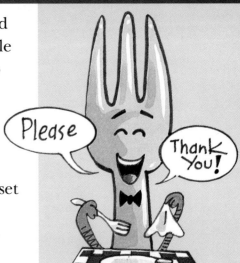

1. Know the correct way to set the table. A neatly set table adds to the enjoyment of eating. Be sure everything is on the table so you do not have to keep getting up to get things.

2. Wash your hands before eating. Other people will see your hands and fingers when you are eating.

3. Place your napkin in your lap. Your napkin collects spills. You can keep foods and beverages from getting on your clothes and on the chair and carpet.

4. Wait until everyone is at the table and served before you begin to eat. It is OK to begin eating if someone who has not been served tells you to do so.

5. Consider the number of people who must eat before you serve yourself. Do not take more than your fair share. After everyone is served, you can serve yourself seconds.

6. Try the different foods being served. Take a small amount of the foods you think you will not like.

7. Take small bites of food and do not eat fast.

8. Keep your mouth closed when you chew your food.

9. Choose appropriate conversation for eating. Do not bring up stressful topics. Do not bring up topics that make eating unpleasant.

10. Thank the person who prepared the food.

Follow a...
Health Behavior Contract

Name: _____ **Date:** _____

Life Skill: I will protect myself and others from germs in foods and beverages.

Effect on My Health: A foodborne illness is an illness caused by eating foods or drinking beverages that contain germs. If I get a foodborne illness, I might have diarrhea, nausea, vomiting, and cramps. I would need to drink plenty of water and liquids. I would need bed rest.

My Plan: I can help prevent foodborne illnesses. I can avoid spoiled foods and beverages. I will take these actions in the next few days.

I will check three stored foods in my refrigerator. I will smell each food and check for discoloration.

	Foods or Beverages	What I Found
1.		
2.		
3.		

I will check the containers of three foods and beverages. I will notice if they are dented, leaking, or bulging.

	Foods or Beverages	What I Found
1.		
2.		
3.		

I will check the expiration date for three foods or beverages.

	Foods or Beverages	What I Found
1.		
2.		
3.		

How My Plan Worked: I will write about what I learned.

Snack Party

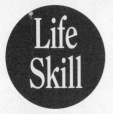

Life Skill

I will use table manners.

Materials: Beverages, snacks, paper cups, paper plates, napkins

Directions: Practice using table manners with classmates.

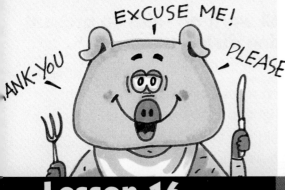

Activity

1. **Plan a snack party.** Set a time with your teacher. Decide what will be served. Decide who will be responsible for bringing beverages, snacks, paper cups, paper plates, and napkins.

2. **Make a list of table manners that will be used at the snack party.** Write this list on the chalkboard.

3. **Make a list of ways to protect classmates from germs in foods and beverages that are served.** Write this list on the chalkboard.

Lesson 16

Review

Vocabulary

Write a separate sentence using each of the vocabulary words listed on page 116.

Health Content

Write answers to the following:

1. How can you keep from eating foods and drinking beverages that are spoiled? **page 117**

2. How can you prepare foods and beverages in a safe way? **page 117**

3. How can you store foods and beverages in a safe way? **page 117**

4. How can you keep from spreading germs when you share foods and beverages? **page 118**

5. What are good table manners you should practice? **page 119**

Step on the Scale: Respect Yourself

Vocabulary

weight management: a plan used to have a healthful weight.

calorie: a unit of energy produced by foods and used by the body.

underweight: a weight below your healthful weight.

overweight: a weight above your healthful weight.

overfat: having too much body fat.

body image: the feeling you have about the way your body looks.

eating disorder: a harmful way of eating because a person cannot cope.

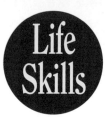

Life Skills

- **I will stay at a healthful weight.**
- **I will work on skills to prevent eating disorders.**

Suppose you step on a scale and read your weight. Would you weigh the right amount for your age, sex, and body frame? Would you be underweight? Overweight? For good health, you need to stay at a healthful weight. Then you will have more energy. You will look and feel your best. When you are older, you will be less likely to have heart disease and certain cancers.

The Lesson Objectives

- Explain how to maintain a healthful weight.
- Explain why it is risky to be overfat.
- Discuss ways to have a positive body image.
- Tell the causes, signs, and treatment for eating disorders.

How Can I Stay at a Healthful Weight?

Weight management is a plan used to have a healthful weight. Weight management is based on calories. A **calorie** is a unit of energy produced by foods and used by the body. You take in calories when you eat food. You use up calories when you are active. The number of calories you take in and use is important. It determines if you stay a healthful weight, gain weight, or lose weight.

Calories in Some Foods

Foods	Amount	Calories
Apple	1	75
Banana	1	130
Cake, chocolate	1 piece	350
Chips	10	150
Cola beverage	12 ounces	150
French fries	10	137
Hamburger on bun	3 ounces	330
Milk, whole	1 cup	159
Popcorn, plain	1 cup	54
Spaghetti	1 cup	140

Calories Used Per Hour

Activity	Calories
Basketball	525
Cycling, 6 mph	300
Desk work	132
Piano playing	140
Running, 6 mph	600
Sitting and reading	72
Sleeping	60
Swimming	300
Walking, 2.5 mph	216

To Stay a Healthful Weight

Suppose you want to stay a healthful weight. Eat the same number of calories from foods as the number of calories you use to be active.

To Gain Weight

Underweight is a weight below your healthful weight. If you are underweight, get checked by a physician. To gain weight, eat more food to take in more calories. Eat more servings of healthful foods. Do not eat more servings of fatty foods. Do not eat more servings of foods with sugar. Choose physical activities that build muscle. More muscle adds weight to your body.

To Lose Weight

Overweight is a weight above your healthful weight. If you are overweight, take in fewer calories from foods. Eat foods that are low in calories. Use up more calories with physical activity.

Balancing Act

Activity

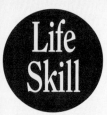

Life Skill

I will stay at a healthful weight.

Materials: Paper, pen or pencil, markers

Directions: Study the illustration. The illustration shows how to stay at a healthful weight. The labels tell you to balance the calories you take in from foods with the calories you use to be active.

1. **Draw an illustration that shows what someone who is underweight should do to gain weight.** Label your illustration.

2. **Draw an illustration that shows what someone who is overweight should do to lose weight.** Label your illustration.

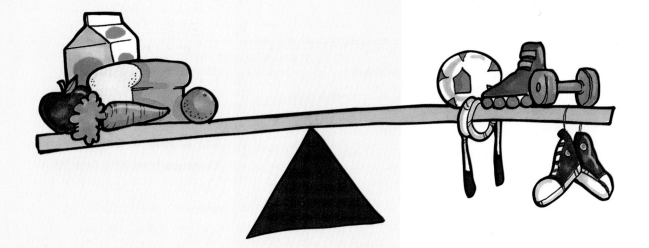

Why Is It Risky to Be Overfat?

Your body is made of two kinds of tissue. There is lean tissue and fat tissue. Your muscles are made from lean tissue. Lean tissue helps you have body tone. Fat tissue is tissue that surrounds and protects body parts. Having a certain amount of body fat tissue is healthful. There is a layer of fat tissue beneath your skin. It acts like a warm coat and keeps you warm in cold weather. When it rains, the fat tissue causes the rain to roll off your skin.

Some people have too much fat tissue. **Overfat** is having too much body fat. You can get overfat if you are overweight. You can get overfat if you are not active. Your muscle will turn to fat tissue. A *couch potato* is a person who is inactive. A couch potato sits on the couch in front of the TV instead of being active. It is risky to be a couch potato and to get overfat. Being overfat increases the risk of heart disease and certain kinds of cancers. Once young people become overfat they are less likely to work out.

How do you know if you are overfat? The best way is to measure body composition. This might be taken if you take a physical fitness test at school. There is another way, too. You can use the pinch test. Pinch a fold of skin on your upper arm. Guess the thickness of the fold of skin. You are overfat if the fold of skin is more than one inch thick.

If you are overfat, check with your doctor. Your doctor can help you make a plan. The plan will include plenty of physical activity. Running, swimming, biking, and skating help reduce body fat.

Walking, skiing, dancing, and playing soccer and basketball also reduce body fat. Your doctor might suggest a weight loss program, too.

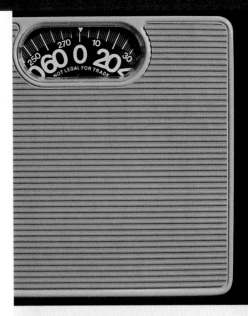

What Happens If You Step on a Scale

Suppose you work out very hard to reduce body fat. You pinch a fold of skin on your upper arm. There is no longer any more than an inch. You have trimmed down. Your abdominal muscles are stronger. You step on a scale to learn how much you weigh. And you weigh more. Why? Muscle tissue weighs more than fat tissue. This is why stepping on a scale does not tell you if you are overfat.

How Can I Develop a Positive Body Image?

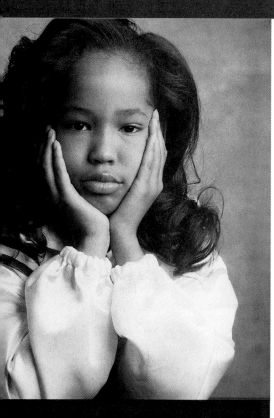

I will work on skills to prevent eating disorders.

Your **body image** is the feeling you have about the way your body looks. Suppose you like and accept the way you look. Then you have a positive body image. Why do you need to have a positive body image? If you do, you are more likely to take care of your body. You are able to resist pressures to harm your body. You do not choose harmful ways to change the way you look.

There are ways to develop a positive body image.

Accept your heredity.

Your heredity influences the way your body looks. Consider the height and body frame of your biological parents. You are likely to be about the same height. Your body frame will be similar, too. Suppose you take after your biological father. He might have a large body frame. Then you are likely to have a large body frame, too. You cannot change your height or body frame.

Accept changes that are happening in your body.

Your body is beginning to change to be more like an adult. It might take time for you to get used to these body changes. For example, you are growing hair under your arms. If you are a girl, your body shape is changing. These body changes are normal. Talk to your parents or guardian if body changes concern you.

Keep a neat and clean appearance.

Wear clean and pressed clothes. Bathe or shower each day. Keep your fingernails clipped and clean. Brush and floss your teeth often. Being well-groomed helps you feel good about yourself.

Do not compare yourself to others.

When you watch television or movies, do not compare yourself to actors or actresses. Do not compare yourself to professional athletes. Do not compare yourself to a classmate who is more popular than you. Remember, you are unique. You are one of a kind.

Be the best you.

You will be second best if you try to be someone you are not.

Do not be critical of the way others look.

One way to accept yourself is to accept others. If you are critical of others, you are more likely to be hard on yourself. Remind your friends that they are unique. Notice when they are well-groomed. Compliment them on the way they look.

Work to develop self-respect.

Self-respect is the good feelings you have about yourself when you behave in responsible ways. Choose responsible actions. Then you will be proud of yourself. Your parents or guardian will be proud of you. You will not be as wrapped up in how you look.

Get plenty of physical activity.

A hard workout is good for your body. Push your body to the max. You will be aware that your muscles have worked. Be aware of your body's performance. This can give you a good feeling.

The Messages in Media

Media are ways of sending messages. Television programs, magazine ads, and radio commercials are kinds of media. You get messages by watching or listening to them. What effect do these messages have on you? Do you compare yourself to children you see on TV or in ads? Remember, you are one of a kind.

What Are the Facts About Eating Disorders?

An **eating disorder** is a harmful way of eating because a person cannot cope. Some young people feel uncomfortable with the body changes that occur at puberty. Some young people cannot express feelings. Some young people do not have self-respect. Some young people compare themselves to movie stars or athletes. They use food to cope. They eat for comfort. Or they do not eat to gain control.

Binge eating disorder is frequently stuffing oneself with food. People stuff themselves when they feel lonely, sad, or angry. People who have this disorder often are overweight.

Bulimia (boo·LEE·mee·uh) is an eating disorder in which a person stuffs himself or herself and then tries to rid the body of food. People who have bulimia stuff themselves when they cannot cope. Then they are upset that they did. They throw up or take laxatives to get rid of what they ate. A laxative is a drug that causes bowel movements.

Anorexia (a·nuh·REK·see·uh) is an eating disorder in which a person starves himself or herself. People who have anorexia feel out of control. They feel they are in control if they do not eat.

Binge eating disorder occurs in teen boys and girls. The other two eating disorders occur mostly in teen girls. The pressure to be thin is a reason some teens have eating disorders. All three eating disorders cause health problems. Stuffing oneself with high-fat and high-calorie foods is harmful. The arteries can get clogged with fat.

What If My Friend Starves or Vomits After Eating?

Young people who have an eating disorder try to make others think they do not. They try to hide their behavior. They make up excuses if a friend calls them on their behavior. Suppose you know someone who starves or who vomits after eating. These are not healthful behaviors. Talk to your parents, guardian, or other trusted adult. Your friend needs help.

Starving oneself is harmful, too. The body does not get the nutrients it needs for growth. Throwing up causes problems with teeth and gums. It harms the digestive system.

Young people who have an eating disorder need medical attention. They need a physical examination and treatment. A hospital stay might be needed. Young people who have an eating disorder need counseling. They need to learn to express feelings. They need to learn to accept their body.

Recovery is a slow and long process. Young people who have an eating disorder can have a relapse. They can get back into the harmful behavior. This happens if they do not stick to their plan. They cannot begin to deny behavior again. They cannot go back to old ways of coping. They must ask for help if they are stressed.

Lesson 17

Review

Vocabulary

Write a separate sentence using each of the vocabulary words listed on page 122.

Health Content

Write answers to the following:

1. How can you stay at a healthful weight? Gain weight? Lose weight? **page 123**
2. Why is it risky to be overfat? **page 125**
3. How can you have a positive body image? **pages 126–127**
4. What are three eating disorders? **page 128**
5. What are some causes of eating disorders? The treatments? **pages 128–129**

Unit 4 Review

Health Content

Review your answers for each Lesson Review in this unit. Write answers to each of the following questions.

1. What minerals does the milk group provide? **Lesson 14 page 104**
2. How many servings do you need each day from the fruit group? **Lesson 14 page 105**
3. What are tips to help you eat fewer fats? **Lesson 14 page 106**
4. How do you know if your food choices are healthful? **Lesson 15 page 112**
5. Why might you blot French fries with a napkin? **Lesson 15 page 114**
6. What are the symptoms for foodborne illness? **Lesson 16 page 117**
7. How do good table manners help you? **Lesson 16 page 119**
8. How do you know if you are overfat? **Lesson 17 page 125**
9. Why do you need to have a positive body image? **Lesson 17 page 126**
10. Why do some people stuff themselves with food? **Lesson 17 page 128**

Multicultural Health

At the grocery store, look for an example of an ethnic food. See how its food label is the same or different from other labels you have seen. Write a paragraph explaining what you found.

Guidelines for Making Responsible Decisions™

Friday there is a party at your school. The outfit you want to wear is a little tight around the waist. A classmate says you can get into your outfit by Friday. Your classmate gives you some laxatives. Your classmate suggests that you starve for the next four days. Use a separate sheet of paper. Answer "yes" or "no" to each of the following questions. Explain each answer.

1. Is it healthful for you to starve and use laxatives?
2. Is it safe for you to starve and use laxatives?
3. Do you follow rules and laws if you starve and use laxatives?
4. Do you show respect for yourself and others if you starve and use laxatives?
5. Do you follow your family's guidelines if you starve and use laxatives?
6. Do you show good character if you starve and use laxatives?

What is the responsible decision to make?

Family Involvement

Help your parents or guardian make their grocery list. Give them a list of five healthful snacks.

Vocabulary

Number a sheet of paper from 1–10. Read each definition. Next to each number on your sheet of paper, write the vocabulary word that matches the definition.

ethnic food	Dietary Guidelines
overfat	fast food restaurant
eating disorder	body image
balanced diet	table manners
calorie	foodborne illness

1. A daily diet that includes the correct number of servings from the food groups in the Food Guide Pyramid. **Lesson 14**
2. A place that serves food quickly. **Lesson 15**
3. Polite ways to eat. **Lesson 16**
4. A food often eaten by a specific culture. **Lesson 15**
5. A unit of energy produced by foods and used by the body. **Lesson 17**
6. Suggested goals for eating to help you stay healthy and live longer. **Lesson 14**
7. Harmful ways of eating because a person cannot cope. **Lesson 17**
8. Too much body fat. **Lesson 17**
9. An illness caused by eating foods or drinking beverages that contain germs. **Lesson 16**
10. The feeling you have about the way your body looks. **Lesson 17**

Health Literacy

Effective Communication

Design a booklet of table manners. Include the table manners that were discussed in Lesson 16. Include at least two more table manners.

Self-Directed Learning

Find a cookbook that contains recipes for ethnic foods. Copy one of the recipes on a sheet of paper. Check the ingredients in the recipe. Check the way the food is prepared— cooked, fried, or broiled. Check the Dietary Guidelines. Decide if the recipe is a healthful one.

Critical Thinking

Suppose you were at a party with friends. There are chips and a bowl of salsa to eat. A friend dips a chip in the salsa and takes a bite. Then he dips the same chip back into the bowl of salsa. Would you take salsa from the bowl? Why or why not?

Responsible Citizenship

Review the Dietary Guidelines. Goal 7 is "Do not drink alcohol." Design a pledge card that reads, "I will not drink alcohol."

Unit 5

Personal Health and Physical Activity

Checking Out Checkups

Vocabulary

physician: a medical doctor who is trained to diagnose and treat illnesses.

medical checkup: a series of tests that measure your health status.

symptom: a change in your behavior or a body function.

nearsighted: having clear vision up close and blurred vision far away.

farsighted: having clear vision far away and blurred vision up close.

hearing loss: the inability to hear or interpret certain sounds.

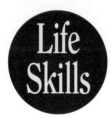

Life Skills

- **I will have regular checkups.**
- **I will help my parents or guardian keep my personal health record.**

Regular checkups provide information about your health status. You learn about your growth. You learn whether your vision and hearing are normal. Checkups help you take action if needed. You can make a plan with your physician to stay healthy.

The Lesson Objectives

- Tell when to have medical checkups.
- List ways to protect your vision.
- List ways to protect your hearing.
- Tell reasons to keep a personal health record.

When Do I Need Medical Checkups?

A **physician** (fuh·ZI·shun) is a medical doctor who is trained to diagnose and treat illnesses. To diagnose means to identify the cause of a symptom. Your relationship with your physician is important. Your physician can help you make a plan to stay healthy. Your physician can answer questions you have about your health.

You need to have a medical checkup each year.

A **medical checkup** is a series of tests that measure your health status. Your physician will check your height and weight. He or she will talk with you about your growth. Your physician will take your blood pressure. He or she will listen to your heart and lungs. You might be asked for a sample of urine and blood. Urine and blood are sent to a lab. They give you information about your health.

You might need a sports checkup if you play sports.

A *sports checkup* is a series of tests you have before you can play sports. Your physician checks to see if there is any reason you should not play. He or she helps you make a plan to play safely. For example, some young people have allergies. Others have asthma. They might need medicines when they play sports. Some young people need special glasses to play.

You need a medical checkup if you have symptoms.

A **symptom** is a change in your behavior or a body function. Tell your parents or guardian if you have symptoms. They will call your physician so you can be checked. Here are symptoms that should be checked:

- Shortness of breath
- Loss of desire to eat
- Blood in your saliva
- Blood in your urine
- Pain when you go to the bathroom
- Coughing that does not go away
- Fever of 100°F or higher for more than a day
- Dizziness
- Swelling of joints
- Bad pain

How Can I Protect My Vision?

Vision is your sight. You might have your vision tested at your school by a nurse or teacher. Vision screening can help discover problems. Signs of vision problems include squinting and leaning forward to see. Another sign is holding a book close in order to read it. Someone with a vision problem might have difficulty reading traffic signs or the chalkboard. This person might need to move close to see. Let your teacher or parent know if you think you have a vision problem.

Even if you do not have signs of vision problems, you need regular eye checkups. You might see a special physician for your eyes. An *optometrist* (ahp·TAH·muh·trist) is a person who is trained to examine eyes and diagnose and treat vision and eye problems. This person cannot prescribe medication. An *ophthalmologist* (ahf·thuh·MAHL·uh·jist) is a physician who studies diseases and disorders of the eye. He or she can prescribe medicine and glasses and perform eye surgery. An *optician* (ahp·TI·shuhn) is a person who grinds lenses and makes glasses.

During an eye exam, the physician does several kinds of eye tests. He or she tests how well you can see close up and far away. **Nearsighted** is having clear vision up close and blurred vision far away. If you are nearsighted, it is hard for you to read the chalkboard. **Farsighted** is having clear vision far away and blurred vision up close. If you are farsighted, it is hard to read a book.

Vision problems can be corrected with glasses, contact lenses, or surgery. *Contact lenses* are lenses that fit directly on the eye for clear vision. There are several kinds of contact lenses. Hard lenses or gas-permeable lenses are made of clear plastic. They are worn during the day and taken out at night. They must be cleaned. Soft lenses absorb water. They are more comfortable than hard lenses. Some soft lenses can be worn for more than 24 hours. Soft lenses also must be kept very clean. Some soft lenses can be thrown away. They are worn only once. They often are worn by people who have allergies.

If you wear contact lenses, pay attention to the instructions for use. Know how to clean and store your lenses. Wash your hands before putting them in or taking them out.

Laser surgery is the newest way to correct vision. A beam of light is used to reshape the eyeball. The surgery is very quick.

Ways to Protect Your Vision

- Do not rub your eyes. You might scratch your eye or get pathogens in your eyes.
- Use your own towel and washcloth. This helps keep you from getting eye infections from someone else.
- Carry sharp objects with the points down.
- Avoid eyestrain. Give your eyes a rest when they feel tired. Read with a light shining from behind your back rather than one shining in your eyes. Keep a light on in the room where you watch TV.
- Wear safety eyeglasses for sports in which you need them.
- Have your vision checked each year.
- Protect your eyes from the sun's rays. Never look directly into the sun. Wear sunglasses when you are in bright sunlight.

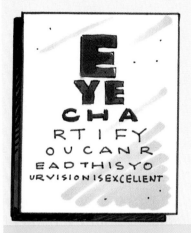

Caution: Choose Sunglasses with Care

Ultraviolet (UV) rays from the sun can damage your eyes. Wear sunglasses to protect your eyes. Suppose you plan to ski in a high altitude. You will be closer to the rays of the sun. Even if it is very cold, you need sunglasses for protection. Suppose it is a warm day and you go swimming. Wear sunglasses by the pool or lake. Water reflects the sun's rays. Choose sunglasses that are dark. Look in the mirror. You should not be able to see your eyes through them. Choose safety sunglasses that do not break. Check to see that the sunglasses protect against both kinds of rays—UVA and UVB.

How Can I Protect My Hearing?

Hearing loss is the inability to hear or interpret certain sounds. Signs of hearing loss might include an earache or a constant buzzing sound. Other signs might include feeling dizzy, asking that questions be repeated, and turning the head to hear.

An *audiologist* (AW·dee·AH·luh·jist) is a person who tests hearing. An *audiometer* (AW·dee·AH·muh·ter) is a machine used to test hearing. The person taking the test wears earphones to hear sounds from the machine. At first, the sound is very soft. Then it becomes louder. The person being tested tells when he or she first hears the sound. The person might have hearing loss if sounds are not heard until they are very loud.

Some people with hearing loss wear a hearing aid. A *hearing aid* is a device that makes sounds louder. It might be worn inside the ear. Sometimes it is put on the frame of a person's glasses.

There are many reasons for hearing loss. The most common are an ear infection, damage to the eardrum, and listening to constant loud noise. You might get an ear infection when pathogens enter and move through the ear. Pathogens also can enter the ear from the throat.

Ways to Protect Your Hearing

- Clean your ears properly. Never put anything inside the ear. The eardrum might become damaged. A physician should remove any wax buildup.
- Protect your eardrum by wearing a safety helmet for certain sports. These sports include football, hockey, baseball, wrestling, bicycling, and in-line skating.
- Protect your ears from loud noises. Do not play the radio or TV too loudly. Be careful when you listen to music while wearing headphones.
- Have your hearing checked each year.
- Blow your nose gently.
- Get treatment for ear infections right away.

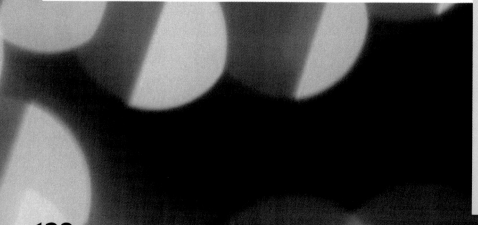

Personal Health Record

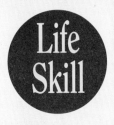

Life Skill

I will help my parents or guardian keep my personal health record.

Materials: Folder, paper, pencil

Directions: A *personal health record* is written information about your health. It is kept in a folder, on the computer, or in another place where you can get it right away. You take this information to your physician when you have a checkup. It helps your physician know about your past. Your physician can help you make a plan to stay healthy. Collect the following information with your parents or guardian. Place it in a folder.

Facts About Your Birth

- Date of your birth and your birth weight
- Name and address of the hospital in which you were born
- Copy of your birth certificate

Facts About Your Family Health History

- Diseases common in your blood relatives
- Age of death of your blood relatives

Facts About Your Health Care

- Dates that you had shots or boosters and for what diseases
- Dates of your most recent medical checkup and dental checkup
- Names of any medicine you take

Activity

Lesson 18

Review

Vocabulary

Write a separate sentence using each of the vocabulary words listed on page 134.

Health Content

Write answers to the following:

1. When do you need to have medical checkups? **page 135**
2. How can vision problems be corrected? **page 137**
3. What are seven ways to protect your vision? **page 137**
4. What are six ways to protect your hearing? **page 138**
5. What are reasons to keep a personal health record? **page 139**

Neatness: An Owner's Manual

Vocabulary

posture: the way you hold your body as you sit, stand, and move.

scoliosis: a curving of the spine to one side of the body.

plaque: a sticky substance on teeth that contains bacteria.

calculus: hardened plaque.

periodontal disease: a disease of the gums and bone that support the teeth.

grooming: taking care of your body and having a neat and clean appearance.

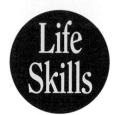

Life Skills

- I will follow a dental health plan.
- I will be well-groomed.

Do you stand with confidence? Do you have a pleasant smile? Are you well-groomed? Grooming and neatness counts. It gives other people an impression of what you are like. It helps you keep your self-respect.

The Lesson Objectives

- Explain how to develop correct posture.
- Make and follow a plan for dental health.
- Discuss ways to care for your skin, hair, and nails.

How Can I Develop Correct Posture?

Your **posture** is the way you hold your body as you sit, stand, and move. Correct posture gives your body organs room to perform. It also allows your blood to flow easily to your organs. Correct posture helps you look and feel good. It can help improve your self-respect. Correct posture prevents backaches.

It is important that you have correct posture. Stand so that you can draw an imaginary straight line through your neck, shoulders, lower back, pelvis and hip, knee, and ankle joints. Sit so that your hips and backs of your thighs support your weight. Keep your feet flat on the floor. Sit in chairs that give support to your lower back.

Use abdominal exercises to develop correct posture. Exercises, such as curl-ups, strengthen your abdominal muscles and prevent them from sagging outward. Stay at a healthful weight.

Scoliosis (skoh·lee·OH·sis) is a curving of the spine to one side of the body. One shoulder or hip might be higher than the other. This curving affects a person's posture. It can affect how the heart, lungs, and nervous system work. Some cases result from muscle diseases. Often, the cause is unknown.

Your school nurse or teacher might check for scoliosis. If this is found, a person should be checked by a physician. The physician might suggest exercises to strengthen back muscles. A back brace might be worn to straighten the spine. People who have a severe case might need surgery.

Flatten Those Abdominal Muscles

Lie with your head, shoulders, back, and buttocks flat on the floor. Bend your knees so that your legs are up and your feet are flat on the floor. Pull in your abdominal muscles as tight as you can. Hold for five seconds. Relax for five seconds. Repeat five times.

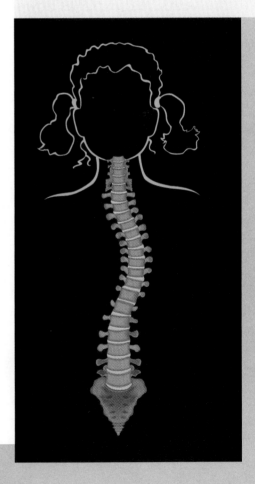

What Can I Include in My Dental Health Plan?

Your teeth should last a lifetime if you care for them. Regular toothbrushing helps remove plaque and food from your teeth. **Plaque** (PLAK) is a sticky substance on teeth that contains bacteria. Plaque is always forming on your teeth, especially near the gum line. Plaque combines with sugar to make acid. The acid can make holes called cavities in the enamel of your teeth.

Your teeth need to be cleaned, polished, and examined every six months. A *dental hygienist* (DEN·tuhl hy·JE·nist) works with a dentist to take care of patients' teeth. This person cleans and polishes teeth, takes X-rays, and explains how to care for teeth and gums.

When your teeth are cleaned, calculus is removed. **Calculus** (KAL·kyuh·luhs) is hardened plaque. If calculus is not removed, the gums can become red and sore. *Gingivitis* (jin·juh·VY·tuhs) is a condition in which the gums are sore and bleed easily. It also can be caused by improper toothbrushing. If this condition worsens, the gums slowly separate from the teeth and make spaces. A dentist will tell a person what to do.

Periodontal (per·ee·oh·DAHN·tuhl) **disease** is a disease of the gums and bone that support the teeth. This disease can begin at your age. It destroys the bone that supports teeth. In time, the teeth become loose.

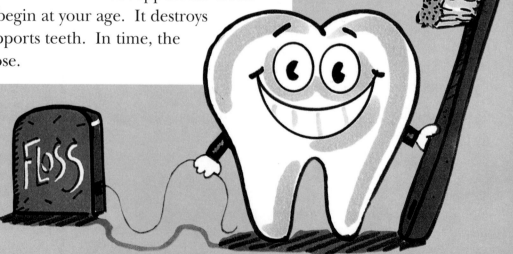

During a dental checkup, your dentist will check to see if your teeth are straight. You might need braces if your teeth are crooked. *Braces* are wires used to move the jaws and teeth. An *orthodontist* (or·thuh·DAHN·tist) is a dentist who is trained to fit braces. Sometimes, teeth must be pulled to make room for teeth being straightened.

Suppose you wear braces. Your orthodontist will give you tips on caring for them. You will need a special mouthguard if you play sports. A mouthguard is something that is worn inside the mouth during sports. It protects the teeth from injury. Your orthodontist also will tell you other ways to protect your braces and teeth. Do not eat hard candies that can break off parts of your braces. Do not eat sticky foods like caramels. It is too hard to remove sticky foods with brushing and flossing.

My Dental Health Plan

- Brush your teeth after every meal.
- Use a toothpaste that contains fluoride. Fluoride is a mineral that hardens tooth enamel.
- Floss at least once a day. *Flossing* is a way to remove plaque and bits of food from between the teeth.
- Flossing helps remove the plaque and food near and under the gumline.
- Choose foods and beverages with calcium. Calcium is a mineral that makes teeth strong.
- Choose foods and beverages with vitamin C. Vitamin C keeps your gums healthy.
- Limit the amount of sugar you eat. Choose foods that are naturally sweet such as an apple.
- Wear a mouthguard for sports.
- Wear a safety belt when riding in a car.
- Have your teeth cleaned and checked every six months.

What Are Ways to Care for My Skin? Hair? Nails?

Grooming is taking care of your body and having a neat and clean appearance. Part of grooming is taking care of your skin, hair, and nails.

There are many glands in your skin. *Perspiration* (per·spuh·RAY·shuhn) is a liquid produced in sweat glands. This liquid leaves the body through tiny openings in the skin called pores. You perspire all the time. Sometimes, perspiration has an odor. Washing with soap and water and using grooming products help prevent this odor. A *deodorant* (dee·OH·duh·ruhnt) is a grooming product used under the arm to control body odor. An *antiperspirant* (an·tee·PUHR·spuh·ruhnt) is a grooming product used under the arms that reduces the amount of perspiration. This product also controls body odor. Both of these products work best when used after a bath or shower.

Sebaceous (si·BAY·shuhs) *glands* are oil glands that produce sebum. *Sebum* (SEE·buhm) is an oily sub-stance that keeps the skin from drying. Sometimes a person's glands produce too much sebum. The skin might become infected. There is swelling and redness. The result is a pimple. *Acne* is a skin disorder in which pores in the skin are clogged with oil. Do not pick or squeeze acne. A doctor can suggest medicine for acne.

Ways to Care for Your Hair

- Shampoo your hair regularly.
- Use a special shampoo if you have dandruff. *Dandruff* is flakes of dead skin cells on the scalp.
- Brush your hair each day to increase blood flow.
- Wear a hat when you are in the sun.
- Do not share a brush, comb, or hat. This can spread head lice. Head lice are insects that lay eggs in the hair.

Ways to Care for Your Nails

- Scrub your nails with a nail brush.
- Trim your finger-nails. Smooth edges with a nail file.
- Clip your toenails straight across.
- Seek prompt attention for an infection.

Ways to Care for Your Skin

- Keep skin clean to avoid body odor.
- Wear a sunscreen with an SPF of at least 15. Use sunscreen 30 minutes before you are in the sun. Reapply often. Use a water repellent sunscreen if you go swimming or boating.

Use... Guidelines for Making Responsible Decisions™

Your friend comes over to ride bikes. It's sunny outside and she has forgotten her hat. She asks if she can wear one of your baseball hats.

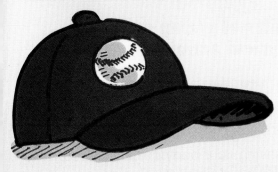

Use a separate sheet of paper. Answer "yes" or "no" to each of the following questions. Explain each answer.

1. Is it healthful to let your friend wear your hat?

2. Is it safe to let your friend wear your hat?

3. Do you follow rules and laws if you let your friend wear your hat?

4. Do you show respect for yourself and others if you let your friend wear your hat?

5. Do you follow your family's guidelines if you let your friend wear your hat?

6. Do you show good character if you let your friend wear your hat?

What is the responsible decision to make?

Lesson 19

Review

Vocabulary

Write a separate sentence using each of the vocabulary words listed on page 140.

Health Content

Write answers to the following:

1. How can you develop correct posture? **page 141**

2. What should you include in your dental health plan? **page 143**

3. What are ways to care for your nails? **page 144**

4. What are ways to care for your skin? **page 144**

5. What are ways to care for your hair? **page 144**

Physical Activity

Vocabulary

physical fitness: having your body in top condition.

health fitness: having the heart, lungs, muscles, and joints in top condition.

fitness skills: skills that can be used during physical activities.

cardiac output: the amount of blood pumped by your heart each minute.

heart rate: the number of times your heart beats each minute.

blood pressure: the force of blood against the artery walls.

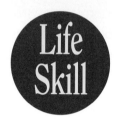

Life Skill

● **I will get plenty of physical activity.**

You need plenty of physical activity to stay healthy. Physical activity helps you gain physical fitness. **Physical fitness** is having your body in top condition. Physical fitness is made up of health fitness and fitness skills.

The Lesson Objectives

● Discuss the benefits of physical activity.

● Describe the kinds of health fitness.

● Describe the kinds of fitness skills.

● Describe five kinds of exercises.

● Explain how aerobic exercises help your heart, blood pressure, and blood vessels.

● Prepare to take a physical fitness test.

What Are the Benefits of Regular Physical Activity?

Physical Activity:

1. **Gives you a healthful appearance.** Physical activity tones muscles. It improves blood flow and gives your skin a healthy glow.

2. **Keeps you from getting stressed out.** Physical activity helps you blow off steam. You relax and sleep better.

3. **Gets you in shape for sports and games.** Physical activity gets your muscles ready for more work. You are ready to play sports and games.

4. **Helps you age in a healthful way.** Physical activity makes your heart and other muscles strong. You stay in shape as you grow older.

5. **Helps you stay at a healthful weight.** Physical activity burns calories. You can eat more food without gaining weight.

6. **Gives you something fun to do with family members and friends.** When you participate, you have fun and get health benefits, too.

7. **Gives you a healthful "high" you cannot get from harmful drug use.** When you work out, your brain releases beta-endorphins. *Beta-endorphins* (BAY·tuh·en·DOR·fuhns) are substances that produce feelings of well-being.

8. **Helps reduce the risk of some diseases when you get older.** Physical activity reduces the risk of having heart disease and some cancers.

9. **Teaches you self-discipline.** *Self-discipline* is the effort you make to do something. You develop self-discipline when you work out often.

10. **Increases the likelihood that you will get good grades.** Studies show that you are more likely to get good grades if you get plenty of physical activity.

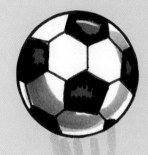

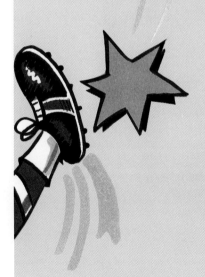

What Are the Five Kinds of Health Fitness?

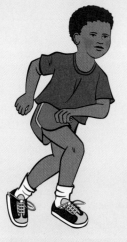

Cardiorespiratory endurance

Health fitness is having the heart, lungs, muscles, and joints in top condition. There are five kinds of health fitness.

- *Muscular strength* is the amount of force your muscles can produce. Your muscles need to be strong to help you lift heavy objects and climb stairs. Strong muscles help you lift, kick, push, and pull.

- *Muscular endurance* is the ability to use the same muscles for a long period of time. You might carry a heavy box to the basement or hold a weight and count to ten.

- *Flexibility* is the ability to bend and move your body easily. You can move your arms and legs in many directions.

- *Cardiorespiratory* (KAR·dee·oh·RES·puh·ruh·TOR·ee) *endurance* is the ability to stay active without getting tired. You are able to run, swim, walk, and bike without becoming tired.

- *Body composition* is the amount of fat tissue and lean tissue in your body. Fat tissue is the stored fat beneath the skin and around the organs. Lean tissue makes up muscles, bones, nerves, skin, and body organs. When you workout regularly, your percent of body fat decreases.

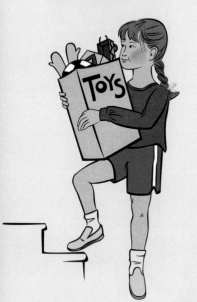

Muscular endurance

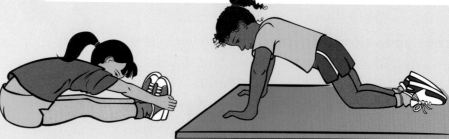

Body composition

Flexibility

Muscular strength

What Are the Six Fitness Skills?

Fitness skills are skills that can be used during physical activities. Fitness skills help you enjoy exercises, sports, and games. They also keep you from being injured as you perform daily activities.

Agility (uh·JI·luh·tee) is the ability to move and change directions. If you are playing soccer, you use agility to change direction to kick the ball. When you use a skateboard, you use agility to move and turn.

Balance is the ability to keep from falling. You use balance to ride your bike, to skateboard, and to rollerblade.

Coordination (KOH·OR·duh·NAY·shuhn) is the ability to use body parts and senses together for movement. For example, when you play basketball, you dribble the ball and run at the same time. Hand-eye coordination is important for many sports and games. If you bat a baseball, your eyes watch the ball as your hands and arms move the bat.

Reaction time is the length of time it takes to move after a signal. Suppose you are going to run a race. A starting gun is fired to signal that the race has begun. When you hear the noise, a message goes to your brain to tell your legs to begin to move. The more quickly you respond, the faster your reaction time.

Speed is the ability to move quickly. You need speed to run a race. You need speed to run bases in a baseball game.

Power is the ability to combine strength and speed. You combine strength and speed to bat a baseball. As power increases, you hit the ball faster and farther.

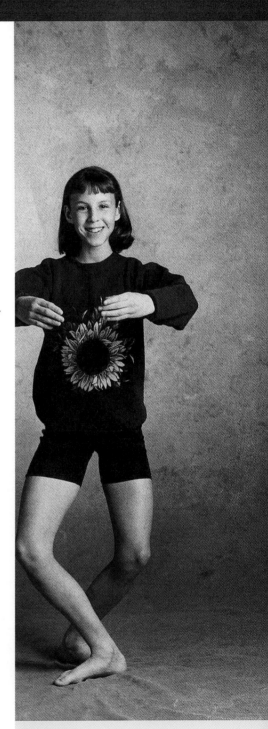

Obstacle Course

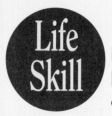

Activity

Life Skill

I will get plenty of physical activity.

Materials: Masking tape, tennis ball, watch with a second hand

Directions: Complete the following activity to use fitness skills you have learned.

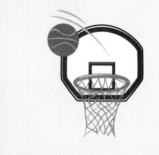

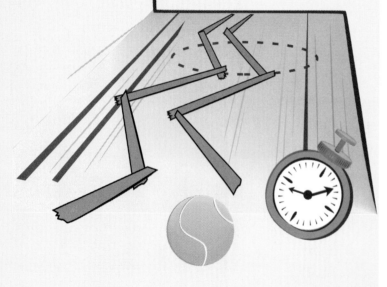

1. **Make an obstacle course.** Clear a large space in your classroom or go outside or to the gym. Use masking tape to make an obstacle course. (See the illustration.) Classmates should line up at the start of the obstacle course.

2. **Show reaction time, agility, and speed.** When your teacher says, "go," move through the obstacle course as fast as you can. Your reaction time is the length of time it takes you to respond when your teacher says "go." Your agility is the ease with which you change directions on the obstacle course. Your speed is how fast you move through the obstacle course.

3. **Show balance.** Move through the obstacle course a second time. This time hop on one foot. Keep your foot on the masking tape. Your balance is your ability to keep from falling or getting too far away from the masking tape.

4. **Show coordination.** Move through the obstacle course again. This time toss the tennis ball up in the air and catch it at the same time as you move. Your coordination is your ability to watch the ball, catch it, and run at the same time.

5. **Show power.** (Complete this step if there is enough space.) Throw the tennis ball as far as you can. Your power is how fast and how far you throw the tennis ball.

What Are Kinds of Exercises I Can Do When I Work Out?

There are five kinds of exercises you can do when you work out. These exercises are as follows.

An *isometric* (eye·suh·ME·trik) *exercise* is an exercise in which you contract your muscles without moving them. These exercises make your muscles larger and stronger. Make a fist and hold it for five seconds. This kind of exercise builds muscle strength.

Isotonic (eye·suh·TAH·nik) *exercise* is an exercise in which you contract muscles to produce movement. Swimming, walking, running, and lifting weights are examples. These exercises help you have muscle strength and endurance.

Isokinetic (eye·suh·ki·NE·tik) *exercise* is an exercise in which weight is moved through a full range of motion. Using an exercise machine with a weight plate is an example. These exercises build strength and help flexibility. Do not use these machines without the supervision of your parents or a guardian.

Anaerobic (an·uhr·OH·bik) *exercise* is exercise that is done for a short time and uses a lot of oxygen. During these exercises, your heart cannot pump blood fast enough to supply the oxygen you need. You become short of breath. Running the 100 meter dash is an example. These exercises help develop muscle strength and endurance. They help develop speed.

Aerobic (uhr·OH·bik) *exercise* is exercise that uses a lot of oxygen for a period of time. During aerobic exercise, you breathe in the same amount of air your body uses. Your heart beats at a steady pace. These exercises lower your percent of body fat. They build cardio-respiratory endurance. Examples include walking fast and bicycling at a steady pace for twenty minutes.

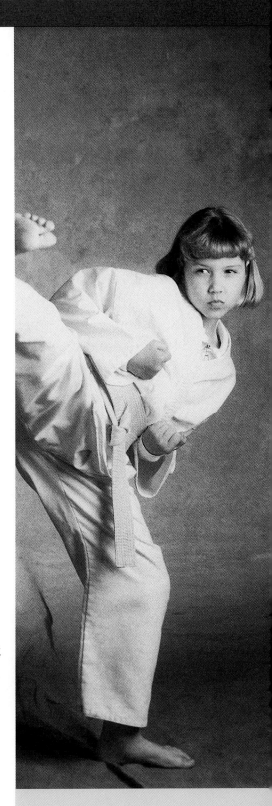

How Does Aerobic Exercise Keep My Heart Healthy?

When you exercise, your muscle cells need more oxygen than usual. Oxygen from the air enters the lungs as you breathe. Blood picks up oxygen as it circulates through the lungs. After leaving the lungs, blood carries oxygen to your muscles, including your heart, and other body cells.

Cardiac output is the amount of blood pumped by your heart each minute. Two actions influence cardiac output. One is your heart rate. **Heart rate** is the number of times your heart beats each minute. The second action is the amount of blood your heart pumps with each beat.

Cardiac output = your heart rate x the amount of blood your heart pumps with each beat.

Suppose you work out often. You choose aerobic exercises. These exercises make your heart muscle strong. A strong heart muscle pumps more blood with each beat than a weak one. Your heart beats less often to supply the same amount of oxygen to cells.

This gives your heart more rest between each beat. You have a lower resting heart rate. Your *resting heart rate* is your heart rate when you are lying down or sitting quietly. You have better cardiorespiratory endurance.

Aerobic exercises strengthen the heart muscle.

If you have a strong heart muscle, your heart will:

- pump more blood per beat;
- beat less often to supply the same amount of oxygen to cells;
- rest longer between beats;
- have a lower resting heart rate.

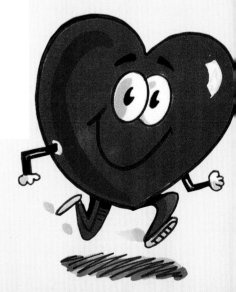

How Does Aerobic Exercise Help My Blood Pressure and Blood Vessels?

Arteries are blood vessels that carry blood away from the heart. Arteries carry blood to all cells in your body. It is easy to remember what the arteries do. Remember the "A." The arteries carry blood away from the heart.

Blood leaves the heart through arteries when your heart beats. **Blood pressure** is the force of blood against the artery walls. Blood pressure keeps your blood moving through your body. Blood pressure forces your blood upward from the lower part of your body and back to your heart.

Being stressed out or overweight can raise your blood pressure. High blood pressure puts more wear and tear on arteries than normal blood pressure. This can damage the arteries and the heart. Regular aerobic exercise lowers resting blood pressure. It keeps fats from sticking to artery walls. Then blood can move more easily through the arteries.

Veins are blood vessels that bring blood from the body cells back to the heart. Flow of blood in the veins is helped in the following ways.

- Blood pressure helps force blood through the veins.
- Valves in the veins keep the blood from flowing backwards.

The actions of leg muscles during exercise squeeze or push against the veins to keep blood from collecting in the legs. This same action moves blood back to the heart. Aerobic exercises such as running strengthen leg muscles. Strong leg muscles help blood flow easily back to the heart.

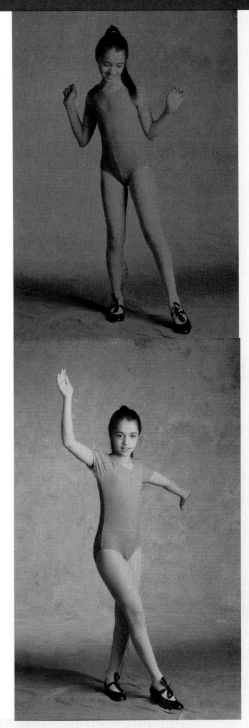

How Can I Prepare to Take Physical Fitness Tests?

There are two tests to measure physical fitness in boys and girls your age. Practice for the test that will be given at your school.

The President's Challenge is a physical fitness test that includes:

- One-mile walk/run
- Curl-ups
- Pull-ups
- V-sit and reach
- Shuttle run

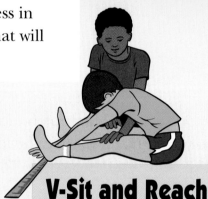

V-Sit and Reach
Measures the flexibility of lower back and calf muscles

President's Challenge

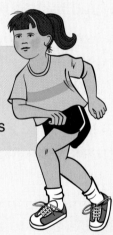

Shuttle Run
Measures strength and endurance of leg muscles

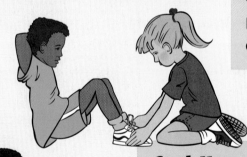

Curl-Ups
Measure strength and endurance of abdominal muscles

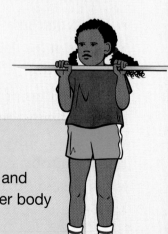

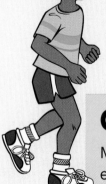

One-Mile Walk/Run
Measures cardiorespiratory endurance

Pull-Ups
Measure strength and endurance of upper body muscles

Prudential FITNESSGRAM

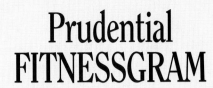

The Prudential FITNESSGRAM is a physical fitness test that includes:

- Percent fat
- One-mile walk/run
- Curl-ups
- Push-ups
- Trunk lift
- Sit and reach

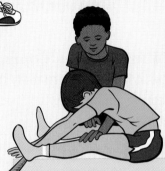

One-Mile Walk/Run

Measures cardiorespiratory endurance

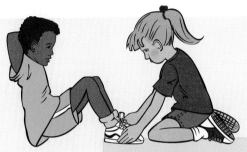

Curl-Ups

Measure strength and endurance of abdominal muscles

Sit and Reach

Measures the flexibility of lower back and calf muscles

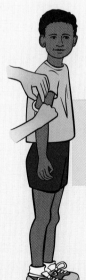

Percent Fat

Measures body composition

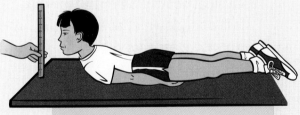

Trunk Lift

Measures strength and flexibility of trunk muscles

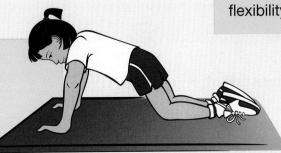

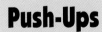

Push-Ups

Measure strength of upper body muscles

Follow a...
Health Behavior Contract

Copy the health behavior contract on a separate sheet of paper.

DO NOT WRITE IN THIS BOOK.

Name:_____ **Date:**_____

Life Skill: I will get plenty of physical activity.

Effect on My Health: Regular physical activity makes my heart muscle strong. It lowers my resting heart rate. It keeps fat from sticking to my arteries. Regular physical activity gives me a healthful appearance. It helps me stay at a healthful weight.

My Plan: I will use a calendar to plan my workouts. I will do the following kinds of exercises.

- Exercises for flexibility on 2–3 days
- Exercises to make muscles strong on 2–4 days
- Aerobic exercises on 3–5 days

I will warm up before I work out. A *warm-up* is three to five minutes of easy physical activity before a workout. This helps me get ready for hard exercise. I will cool down after I work out. A *cool-down* is five to ten minutes of easy exercise after a workout.

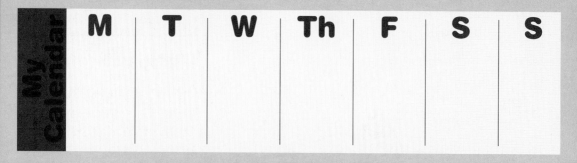

My Calendar	M	T	W	Th	F	S	S

How My Plan Worked: (Complete after one week.)

What Is FITT?

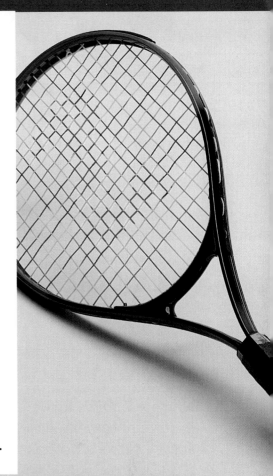

The *FITT formula* is a formula that tells you how to get fitness benefits from your workouts. The formula has four things you must do to have fitness. It is easy to remember the FITT formula. Remember what each of the letters F-I-T-T stands for.

F is for frequency. Make sure you work out frequently. Get a good workout on five different days of the week.

I is for intensity. Make sure your workout is intense or hard enough to get benefits. A trainer, coach, or other adult can help you with this.

T is for time. Make sure your workout is long enough to get benefits. For example, you must do aerobic exercises for at least twenty minutes.

T is for type. Make sure you choose the right types of exercises to get fitness benefits. For example, stretching exercises are right if you want flexibility. But they do not help your cardiorespiratory endurance.

Lesson 20

Review

Vocabulary

Write a separate sentence using each of the vocabulary words listed on page 146.

Health Content

Write answers to the following:

1. What are the benefits of physical activity? **page 147**
2. What are the five kinds of health fitness? **page 148**
3. What are six fitness skills? **page 149**
4. What are five kinds of exercises you can do when you work out? **page 151**
5. How do aerobic exercises help your heart? Your blood pressure? Your blood vessels? **pages 152–153**

Being a Safe and Good Sport

Vocabulary

good sport: a person who respects others and follows safety rules for sports.

warm-up: three to five minutes of easy physical activity before a workout.

target heart rate: a fast and safe heart rate for workouts to get cardiorespiratory endurance.

cool-down: five to ten minutes of easy exercise after a workout.

sprain: an injury to the tissue that connects bones to a joint.

RICE treatment: a treatment for injuries to muscles and bones.

muscle strain: an overstretch of a muscle.

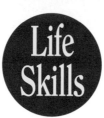

Life Skills

- I will follow safety rules for sports and games.
- I will prevent injuries during physical activity.

Participate in physical activity to the max! Get involved in sports and games. Join a team. Enjoy competing with yourself to get better scores or skills. Enjoy competing with others. Play fair and develop quality relationships with others. At the same time, stay safe. Follow rules. Know how to prevent and treat injuries.

The Lesson Objectives

- Describe actions that show you are a good sport.
- Discuss guidelines for a safe workout.
- Explain how to prevent and treat sprains and strains.

What Are Ways I Can Show I Am a Good Sport?

Suppose you play sports. You might be on a baseball or soccer team. You might be on the swim team for your school or for a club. When you play sports, be a good sport. A **good sport** is a person who respects others and follows safety rules for sports.

There are ways to show you are a good sport.

Play by the rules. Rules for sports help keep order. When players know what is expected, there are fewer injuries. There is less disagreement. Rules give players the same chance to win. No one or no team has an advantage over the other.

Give your best effort. Do what is expected of you. Show up for practice on time. Work hard to learn the skills that you need for the sport that you play. Always try your best whether you or your team is winning or losing. When you give your best effort, you keep your self-respect. Other people respect you.

Do not start fights or join in on fights. Do not say or do anything to start a fight. For example, do not call someone a name or elbow someone. Even if you get away with it, these actions are wrong. Suppose a fight begins between other players. Do not join in. Let an official, referee, or your coach settle disagreements.

Keep a healthful attitude about winning and losing. No one likes to lose. But in a sports event there is a winner and a loser. Sometimes you will be the winner and sometimes you will be the loser. In both cases, recognize your good efforts. Recognize the efforts of other players on your team and on the other team. If you have just lost, think of ways to improve your play. Do not get down on yourself or other players.

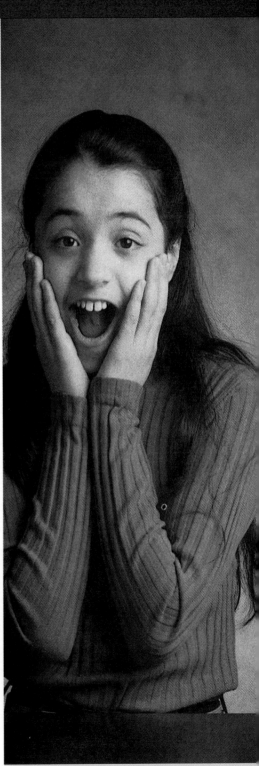

What Are Guidelines for a Safe Workout?

There are guidelines to keep you healthy and safe during a workout.

Choose physical activities that are right for you.
Consider your age, size, and physical condition. If you have a special condition such as asthma, a physician can tell you safe ways to work out.

Use all of the recommended safety equipment.
Be certain that the equipment fits you as it should and is in good condition.

Wear clothing that is appropriate for the weather conditions. During hot weather, wear light colored clothing that breathes. During cold weather, wear layers of clothing. Wear a hat and gloves to stay warm.

Drink fluids before, during and after physical activity. Drink at least eight ounces of water thirty minutes before a workout. Keep replacing fluids during your workout. Do not wait until you are thirsty.

Begin your workout with a warm-up. A **warm-up** is three to five minutes of easy physical activity before a workout. Do slow muscle stretches. Walk or run slowly to gradually increase your heart rate.

Perform aerobic exercises at your target heart rate. Your **target heart rate** is a fast and safe heart rate for workouts to get cardiorespiratory endurance. A doctor or coach can advise you what your target heart rate should be.

End your workout with a cool-down. A **cool-down** is five to ten minutes of easy exercise after a workout. During cool-down your heart rate slows.

Remember to Use Safety Equipment

- Bicycle safety helmet
- Safety eyeglasses
- Mouthguard
- Knee brace
- Football helmet
- Batter's helmet
- Shin guard
- Hockey glove

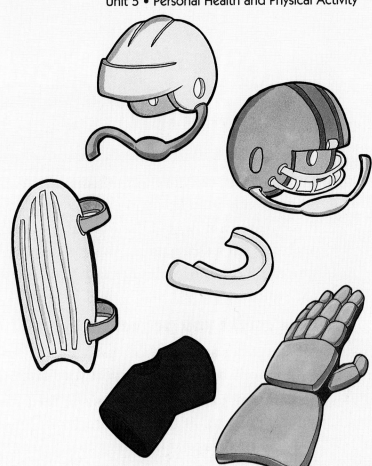

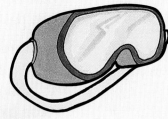

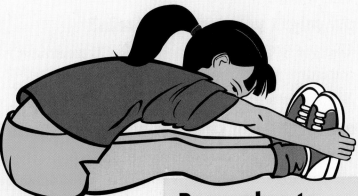

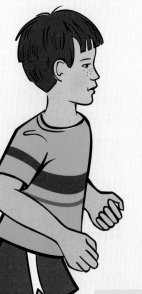

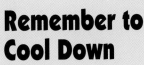

Remember to Cool Down

- Do five to ten minutes of easy exercise. This slows the heart rate. It helps blood from the legs to return to the heart.

Remember to Warm Up

- Do slow muscle stretches to get your muscles ready to do more work.

How Do I Prevent and Treat Sprains and Strains?

A **sprain** is an injury to the tissue that connects bones to a joint. Have you ever sprained an ankle? If you have, you twisted the joint at the ankle. You probably felt a sharp pain. Your ankle became very sore and began to swell. Perhaps you have sprained your knee.

How might you prevent a sprain?

- Select your athletic shoes carefully. High-top athletic shoes can be worn to support your ankles.
- Be on the lookout for changes in the surface of a road or track. If there is a crack or pothole, you might turn your ankle.
- Talk to a coach or your parents or guardian about taping a weak ankle.
- Wear an ankle, knee, or wrist brace if a doctor has told you to.

How might you treat a sprain?

- Use the RICE treatment. The **RICE treatment** is a treatment for injuries to muscles and bones.
- See a doctor if swelling and soreness continue.

How might you prevent a muscle strain?

Have you ever felt a snap and a sharp pain when you were working out? Perhaps you were running and felt a pull in your calf muscles. A **muscle strain** is an overstretch of a muscle.

- Begin your workout with a warm-up of slow stretches.
- Continue your warm-up with walking or slow jogging.

The RICE Treatment

- **R**est the injured part of the body.
- **I**ce the injury with a cold compress or ice pack.
- **C**ompress or wrap the injury with a bandage to stop bleeding. Do not wrap it too tightly. Keep it wrapped for 30 minutes. Then place ice on it for 15 minutes. Then wrap it again for 30 minutes. Repeat this for three hours.
- **E**levate or keep the injured area propped up. This drains the blood and fluid from the injured area.

Recipe for a Winner

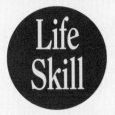

I will follow safety rules for sports and games.

Materials: Paper and pen; colored pencils or marker (optional); computer (optional); one three-ring notebook for the class

Directions: Read the Recipe for a Winner. Choose five of your own ingredients and create your own recipe. Place your recipe in a three-ring notebook with the recipes of your classmates. Use 8 1/2" by 11" paper. Design your recipe on a computer if one is available.

Recipe for a Winner

- Three cups of hard practice
- Four ounces of positive attitude
- Three spoons of self-discipline
- Half pound of sportsmanship
- Pound of character

Activity

Lesson 21

Review

Vocabulary

Write a separate sentence using each of the vocabulary words listed on page 158.

Health Content

Write answers to the following:

1. What are ways you can show that you are a good sport? **page 159**
2. What are guidelines for a safe workout? **page 160**
3. How can you prevent sprains? **page 162**
4. How can you prevent strains? **page 162**
5. How do you use the RICE treatment? **page 162**

Catch Some ZZZs...Sleep

Vocabulary

rest: a period of relaxation.

sleep: deep relaxation in which you are not aware of what is happening around you.

sleep cycle: the stages your body goes through while you sleep.

REM: the stage of sleep when you dream.

cat nap: a 20 to 30 minute nap during the day.

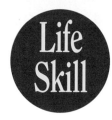

Life Skill

● **I will get enough rest and sleep.**

Rest is a period of relaxation. **Sleep** is deep relaxation in which you not aware of what is happening around you. You need periods of rest during your busy day. You need ten to eleven hours of sleep.

The Lesson Objectives

● Explain what happens during the sleep cycle.

● Discuss reasons why you need sleep.

● Explain how to get enough rest and sleep.

Why Do I Need Rest and Sleep?

The **sleep cycle** is stages your body goes through while you sleep. There are five stages.

Stage 1: Your muscles begin to relax. Tension slowly leaves your body.

Stage 2: Your heart rate slows down by about ten to fifteen beats per minute. You take fewer breaths each minute.

Stage 3: Your blood pressure lowers. Your body temperature lowers.

Stage 4: You go into deep sleep and are very difficult to wake up.

Stage 5: Brain wave activity increases. You begin the REM stage of sleep. **REM** is the stage of sleep when you dream. REM stands for rapid eye movement. While you dream, your eyes dart back in forth in rapid motion. Your brain is as sharp as when you are not asleep. This is why many people try to remember their dreams. During dreams, you are thinking about actions and your life. Your parents or guardian can discuss your dreams with you.

It takes about 90 minutes to go through the stages of sleep. After the REM stage, the sleep cycle begins again. Throughout the night, you repeat the sleep cycle. Suppose someone tries to wake you up or the telephone rings. Your reaction will depend upon which stage of the sleep cycle you are in.

There are good reasons to get plenty of rest and sleep.

- **Rest and sleep protect your health.** During sleep, growth hormone is released. When you sleep, you grow. Body cells are repaired. Your body organs get rest. Your body gets rest so it can fight pathogens and keep you from getting sick.

- **Rest and sleep help you stay in a good mood.** You might get grouchy if you are too tired.

- **Rest and sleep help you have a healthful appearance.** You will appear rested and sharp. Your eyes and skin will have a healthful glow.

- **Rest and sleep help you perform well in school.** You are able to think clearly.

How Do I Get Enough Rest and Sleep?

You can make a plan to get short periods of rest during your busy day.

Tips to Help You Rest and Relax

- **Choose something to help you rest and relax at recess.** Suppose you are very tense. Something active might relax you. Suppose you feel very tired. Perhaps you need to put your head down on your desk for a few minutes.

- **Plan some quiet time for yourself.** Listen to music that relaxes you. Read a book that you enjoy. Take time for a hobby.

- **Take a cat nap.** A **cat nap** is a 20 to 30 minute nap during the day. A cat nap can refresh you. Don't take a long nap because that can interfere with getting a good night's sleep.

- **Plan physical activity that reduces tension.** You use up a lot of energy when your muscles are tense. Try walking or breathing exercises to release tension.

Tips to Help You Get a Good Night's Sleep

- **Give yourself 15 minutes to unwind before you go to sleep.** During this time, do something relaxing. Listen to music. Take a warm bath.

- **Don't go to bed mad or upset.** Work through upset feelings first. Talk to your parents or guardian. Write about upset feelings in a diary or journal.

- **Drink warm milk.** It might help you feel sleepy.

- **Watch what you eat and drink before you go to bed.** Being very full or eating spicy foods can keep you awake. Foods and beverages with caffeine can keep you awake. If you have a full bladder, you will wake up in the night to go to the restroom.

Get Rid of That Tension

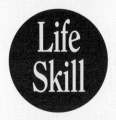

Life Skill
I will get enough rest and sleep.

Materials: None

Directions: Follow the steps at the right to reduce tension. This helps you relax.

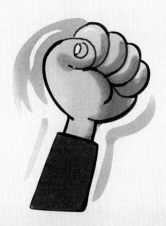

Activity

1. **Make a fist as hard as you can.** Hold the fist for five seconds. Slowly relax your fist.
2. **Tense the muscles in your face.** Keep your face muscles tensed for five seconds. Slowly relax your face muscles.
3. **Pull your abdomen in as tight as possible.** Pretend you will touch your navel to your backbone. Hold this position for five seconds. Slowly relax the muscles in your abdomen.
4. **Curl your toes as tight as possible.** Hold this position for five seconds. Slowly let your toes uncurl.
5. **Share with classmates how you feel after tensing and relaxing muscles.**

Lesson 22

Review

Vocabulary

Write a separate sentence using each of the vocabulary words listed on page 164.

Health Content

Write answers to the following:

1. How much sleep do you need? **page 164**
2. What happens during the sleep cycle? **page 165**
3. What are four reasons you need rest and sleep? **page 165**
4. What are tips to help you rest and relax? **page 166**
5. What are tips to help you get a good night's sleep? **page 166**

Unit 5 Review

Health Content

Review your answers for each Lesson Review in this unit. Write answers to the following questions.

1. Why do you need a checkup before you play on a sports team? **Lesson 18 page 135**

2. What are signs that you might have a vision problem? **Lesson 18 page 136**

3. What are two causes of gingivitis? **Lesson 19 page 142**

4. Why do you need to have calcium in your daily diet? **Lesson 19 page 143**

5. Why do you get a healthful high when you workout? **Lesson 20 page 147**

6. How do regular workouts affect your percent of body fat? **Lesson 20 page 148**

7. What are ways to keep a healthful attitude about winning when you play sports? **Lesson 21 page 159**

8. What should you do if you sprain your ankle? **Lesson 21 page 162**

9. How does rest and sleep protect your health? **Lesson 22 page 165**

10. What should you do if you feel mad or upset at bedtime? **Lesson 22 page 166**

Guidelines for Making Responsible Decisions™

You are playing for a soccer club. You have forgotten your mouthguard for today's game. Your coach does not notice. Use a separate sheet of paper. Answer "yes" or "no" to each of the following questions. Explain each answer.

1. Is it healthful to play soccer without wearing a mouthguard?

2. Is it safe to play soccer without wearing a mouthguard?

3. Do you follow rules and laws if you play soccer without wearing a mouthguard?

4. Do you show respect for yourself and others if you play soccer without wearing a mouthguard?

5. Do you follow your family's guidelines if you play soccer without wearing a mouthguard?

6. Do you show good character if you play soccer without wearing a mouthguard?

What is the responsible decision to make?

Family Involvement

Plan to participate in a physical activity with members of your family. Begin by brainstorming a list of five physical activities. Then select one that everyone would enjoy.

Vocabulary

Number a sheet of paper from 1–10. Read each definition. Next to each number on your sheet of paper, write the vocabulary word that matches the definition.

symptom	target heart rate
good sport	farsighted
cat nap	REM
plaque	scoliosis
health fitness	cardiac output

1. A sticky substance on teeth that contains bacteria. **Lesson 19**
2. Having the heart, lungs, muscles, and joints in top condition. **Lesson 20**
3. A person who respects others and follows safety rules for sports. **Lesson 21**
4. A fast and safe heart rate for workouts to get cardiorespiratory endurance. **Lesson 21**
5. A change in your behavior or a body function. **Lesson 18**
6. A 20 to 30 minute nap during the day. **Lesson 22**
7. The amount of blood pumped by your heart each minute. **Lesson 20**
8. Having clear vision far away and blurred vision up close. **Lesson 18**
9. The stage of sleep when you dream. **Lesson 22**
10. A curving of the spine to one side of the body. **Lesson 19**

Health Literacy

Effective Communication

Make a list of five questions you would like to ask your physician or dentist. Take these questions with you the next time you have a checkup.

Self-Directed Learning

Get permission from your parents or guardian. Go to a drug store and check out the grooming products. Make a list of ten grooming products you find and their cost. Put a plus (+) next to the grooming products you think are necessary.

Critical Thinking

Write a paragraph telling why it is best not to eat pizza right before you go to bed.

Responsible Citizenship

Get permission from your parent or guardian to take part in a run or walk for charity. Ask them to go with you.

Multicultural Health

Check out books from your library that contain pictures of young people from different cultures. Share the pictures with your classmates. Notice how it is important to smile in all cultures.

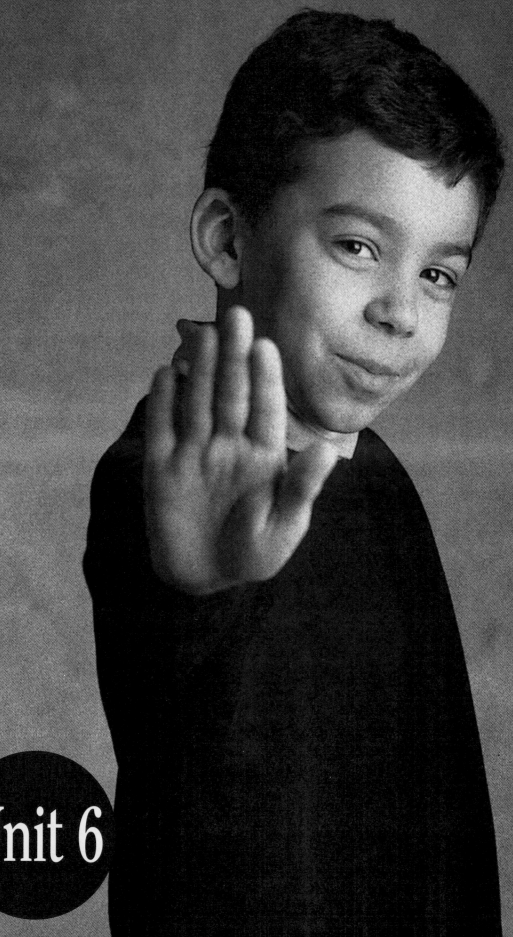

Unit 6

Alcohol, Tobacco, and Other Drugs

Expert Witness... Against Drugs

Vocabulary

drug: a substance that changes the way your body or mind works.

prescription drug: a medicine that you can buy only if a doctor writes an order.

over-the-counter (OTC) drug: a medicine that you can buy without a doctor's order.

drug misuse: the unsafe use of a legal drug that is not on purpose.

drug abuse: the use of an illegal drug or the harmful use of a legal drug on purpose.

drug addiction: a strong desire to take drugs even though drug use causes harm.

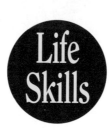

Life Skills

- I will use over-the-counter (OTC) and prescription drugs in safe ways.
- I will tell ways to get help for someone who uses drugs in harmful ways.

A **drug** is a substance that changes the way your body or mind works. A *medicine* is a drug used to prevent, treat, or cure a health condition. A **prescription drug** is a medicine that you can buy only if your doctor writes an order. An **over-the-counter (OTC) drug** is a medicine that you can buy without a doctor's order. It also is called an OTC drug. You need to have facts about drugs to protect yourself and those around you.

The Lesson Objectives

- Discuss responsible drug use.
- Discuss the safe use of prescription and OTC drugs.
- Discuss why you need to recognize drug abuse.
- List steps that lead to drug dependence.
- Tell how to get help for someone who abuses drugs.

What Is Responsible Drug Use?

You will make many decisions today and in the future. The decisions you make about drugs will affect your health and safety. They will affect the health and safety of others. They will reflect your character. Most of your decisions about drugs will be easy to make. Other decisions will be more difficult. At times, your peers will try to influence you.

Most of your peers want you to stay drug-free. They know that drugs should be used to promote health. They do not want you to use drugs for other reasons. If they care about you, they want you to protect your health. They do not want you to break laws or harm those around you.

Some of your peers will pressure you to use drugs in harmful ways. They pressure you to risk your health and safety. They pressure you to risk your future. These peers do not care about what happens to you.

These peers are concerned about themselves. They want you to go along with their wrong decisions. Then they will have support for what they do. Part of being responsible is pointing out to others that you do not support wrong decisions. This puts the pressure on your peers to make responsible decisions.

The lessons in this unit give you the facts and skills you need to make decisions. The rest is up to you. Protect your health and safety. Protect your surroundings. Show that you have character. Always decide on responsible drug use.

Responsible Drug Use for Me Means...

- using prescription drugs correctly.
- using OTC drugs correctly.
- NOT using beverages that contain alcohol.
- NOT using tobacco— it contains nicotine.
- NOT inhaling fumes from products such as glue to get high.
- NOT using illegal drugs, such as marijuana, cocaine, crack, heroin, or amphetamines.

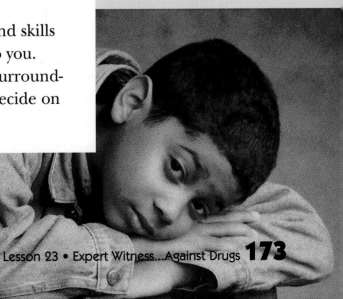

What Are Safe Ways to Use Prescription Drugs?

A prescription drug is a medicine that you can buy only if your doctor writes an order. Dentists and doctors can write orders for prescription drugs. A pharmacist looks at the order and gets the drug for you. There are safe ways to use prescription drugs.

Tell your doctor and your pharmacist if you are taking any other drugs. Taking more than one drug at the same time might not be safe. One drug can change the actions of another drug.

Take prescription drugs only from your parents or guardian or a person of whom they approve. Your parents or guardian are in charge of your medical care.

Follow the directions for taking the drug. The label on the drug will tell the dose. The dose is the amount of the drug you should take. The label will tell you how often to take the drug. The label will say when it is best for you to take the drug. For example, it might say to take the drug with food.

Do not take more than the correct dose. Suppose one pill every six hours is the dose. Do not take more. You might overdose. An overdose is an amount over the correct dose and that can harm health.

Report side effects right away. A side effect is an unwanted reaction to a drug. Your doctor might warn you about side effects. Your pharmacist might give you a sheet that tells side effects. Tell a trusted adult right away if you have side effects.

Do not take another person's prescription drug. The doctor wrote the order for you only.

Keep prescription drugs in their original containers. The original container has the directions for safe use on it.

Drug Interactions

A drug interaction is the effect a drug has on another drug that is taken. Suppose you are taking a drug you got from a doctor. You are injured playing soccer and go to an emergency care facility. You do not tell the doctor who sees you about the drug. The doctor prescribes another drug. You take both drugs. The first drug might make the effects of the second drug much stronger. This can harm your health.

Brand Names vs. Generic Names

Suppose your parent or guardian is buying a prescription drug for you. They might buy a brand name or a generic name. A brand name drug has a registered name or trademark. "Generic" means the drug is not protected by trademark. It has the same ingredients as does a brand name drug.

What Are Safe Ways to Use OTC Drugs?

An over-the-counter, or OTC, drug is a medicine you can buy without a doctor's order. Some common OTC drugs are aspirin, cold tablets, nasal spray, sinus medication, and skin ointment. OTC drugs can be helpful in relieving minor symptoms of an illness.

Use OTC drugs only if they are given to you by your parents or guardian or a person of whom they approve. Your parents or guardians are in charge of your medical care. They decide who can give you medicine if they are unavailable when you need it.

Do not take an OTC drug for any longer than the directions say. You might have a more serious health problem than you think. The OTC drug might make it seem less serious. Then you might put off seeing a doctor. The condition you have might worsen. It might be more difficult to treat because you waited so long.

Stop taking an OTC drug if you have side effects. The label tells you about possible side effects. You might have side effects that are not mentioned on the label. Tell a trusted adult about side effects right away. The adult will call a doctor and ask what to do.

Keep all OTC drugs in their original containers. The original container has the directions for safe use on it.

Do not use an OTC drug past the expiration date. An expiration date is stamped on the container. The drug might not be safe to take after this date. The effects of the drug might be greater or lessened.

Tamper-Resistant Seal

OTC drugs come with a tamper-resistant seal. A *tamper-resistant seal* is an unbroken seal to show a container has not been opened. Do not use an OTC drug if the tamper-resistant seal is broken or missing.

Why Do I Need to Recognize Drug Abuse?

You have just learned safe ways to use prescription and OTC drugs. Suppose you forgot and skipped a dose of your prescription medicine. **Drug misuse** is the unsafe use of a legal drug that is not on purpose. But suppose you took someone else's painkillers on purpose. Suppose you smoked a cigarette. This is drug abuse. **Drug abuse** is the use of an illegal drug or the harmful use of a legal drug on purpose.

There are reasons you need to know about drug abuse.

- To keep from abusing drugs
- To protect yourself from people who abuse drugs
- To get help for someone you care about who abuses drugs
- To follow laws and protect those around you

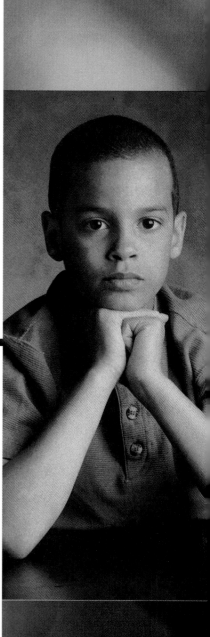

Do You Know Drug Abuse When You See It?

Drug abuse is...

- **Drinking alcohol at a party**
- **Inhaling glue to get high**
- **Taking steroids to bulk up**
- **Taking someone else's prescription medicine**
- **Taking a prescription medicine after your doctor told you to stop taking it**
- **Snorting cocaine just once**
- **Taking a higher dose of a painkiller than your doctor prescribed for you**
- **Chewing smokeless tobacco**

What Are Steps That Lead to Drug Dependence?

An *addiction* is a strong desire to do something even though it is harmful. There are many kinds of addictions. Suppose a person watched TV all the time. As a result, she did not do homework or household chores. She neglected friends. She would have TV addiction. She watched TV even though it affected her life in harmful ways. You probably know of other addictions: shopping addiction, gambling addiction, and so on.

Drug addiction is a strong desire to take drugs even though drug use causes harm. A person who has drug addiction depends on a drug. This is where the term drug dependence comes from. *Drug dependence* is depending on drugs for their emotional or physical effects.

Emotional dependence Some young people use drugs to cope with emotions. Suppose a young male feels insecure. He drinks a few sips of beer to get his courage up. He finds it easier to talk to others when he has been drinking. He depends on drinking rather than on social skills. He has emotional dependence on alcohol.

Physical dependence Some young people get hooked on drugs for their physical effects. Suppose a young female takes painkillers for an injury. Her doctor tells her to stop taking them. But she buys them on the street. She gets used to the effects they have on her body. *Tolerance* is a condition in which more of a drug is needed to get the same effects. If she stops taking the drug, she has withdrawal symptoms. *Withdrawal symptoms* are unpleasant reactions when a drug is no longer taken. Symptoms are nausea, vomiting, shaking, and sweating. She keeps taking the painkillers so she does not have unpleasant reactions. She has physical dependence.

Steps to Drug Dependence

Step 1: A person uses a drug for no health reason.

Step 2: A person uses the drug again and again.

Step 3: A person uses the drug to help deal with emotions or social situations. A person uses more of the drug to get the same effects (tolerance).

Step 4: A person depends on the drug to cope or to relate to others (emotional dependence). A person depends on the drug to stop withdrawal symptoms (physical dependence).

How Can I Get Help for Someone Who Abuses Drugs?

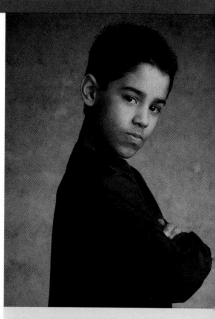

Someone who abuses drugs needs help. A person who abuses a drug even one time needs help. Suppose you smoke a cigarette just once. A friend who knows should speak up and say something to you. Suppose you take another person's prescription drug. A brother or sister should say something to your parents or guardian.

Suppose you are with a friend who sniffs glue. You must tell your friend this is drug abuse. Suppose you are with a friend who sneaks a sip of beer. You must speak up and tell your friend this is drug abuse.

Talk to a trusted adult if you or someone you know abuses drugs. Suppose you have abused a drug. Ask for help. Talk to your parents or guardian. Talk to a teacher, counselor, or member of the clergy. Adults want to guide you and protect you.

Suppose someone you know abuses a drug. You are not squealing if you tell. You are protecting this person and those around you. Talk to a trusted adult who can help this person.

Know that treatment is available. Health care is available for people who abuse drugs. Some people who abuse drugs need medical care. They might need to stay in a hospital or other facility while they get drugs out of their bodies.

The family members and friends learn to set limits. They learn honest talk. They speak about ways they have been harmed by the drug dependence of another person.

Know that people who are drug dependent also need counseling. A counselor helps them learn coping skills. They learn not to depend on drugs. A counselor might work with family members and friends.

Do Not Ignore Signs of Drug Abuse.

- Lying about drug use
- Getting into trouble
- Hanging out with those who use drugs
- Having a sloppy appearance
- Having slurred speech
- Having glassy eyes
- Joining a gang
- Getting in fights
- Showing no interest in activities

Use... Guidelines for Making Responsible Decisions™

A classmate has a family member with depression. The family member takes prescription medicine. Your classmate tells you the medicine will lift your spirits. She gives you two pills.

?

Use a separate sheet of paper. Answer "yes" or "no" to each of the following questions. Explain each answer.

1. Is it healthful for you to take someone else's medicine?
2. Is it safe for you to take someone else's medicine?
3. Do you follow rules and laws if you take someone else's medicine?
4. Do you show respect for yourself and others if you take someone else's medicine?
5. Do you follow your family's guidelines if you take someone else's medicine?
6. Do you show good character if you take someone else's medicine?

What is the responsible decision to make?

Lesson 23

Review

Vocabulary

Write a separate sentence using each of the vocabulary words listed on page 172.

Health Content

Write answers to the following:

1. What is responsible drug use? **page 173**
2. What are safe ways to use prescription drugs? OTC drugs? **pages 174–175**
3. Why do you need to know about drug abuse? **page 176**
4. What are steps that lead to drug dependence? **page 177**
5. How can you get help for someone who abuses drugs? **page 178**

Drug-Free... You and Me!

Vocabulary

drug-free: to say NO to all harmful drug use.

honest talk: the open sharing of feelings.

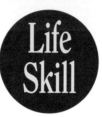
Life Skill

• **I will say NO if someone offers me a harmful drug.**

You can promise to be drug-free. To be **drug-free** is to say NO to all harmful drug use. You keep harmful drugs out of your body. For example, you do not drink or use tobacco. You only use prescription and OTC drugs in safe ways. You stay out of situations in which there will be drug use. You do not go to parties where there will be drugs. You do not sit in the smoking section of a restaurant. You expect other people to be drug-free.

The Lesson Objectives

● List ten reasons to stay drug-free.

● Discuss why you should expect others to be drug-free.

● Tell how to use honest talk with someone who uses harmful drugs.

● Tell ways to say NO if you are pressured to abuse drugs.

● Tell how to say NO to drugs firmly.

What Are Ten Reasons to Be Drug-Free?

Suppose someone asks you why you are drug-free. Here are ten reasons you can give.

1. **I want to obey laws.** I know laws were made to protect me and others. I want to show I respect the law and the police who make sure people follow laws.

2. **I want to follow my parents' or guardian's guidelines.** My parents or guardians trust me. They count on me to be responsible. I do not want to disobey them. I do not want to let them down.

3. **I want to protect my safety.** Drugs can change the way I respond. I do not want to have accidents.

4. **I want to be in control of my actions.** Drugs can change the way I think and feel. I might say or do something I regret later.

5. **I want to be a good example for others.** I have younger brothers and sisters. Or I know younger children I care about. They look up to me. I do not want them to copy wrong behavior.

6. **I want to reduce crime.** Drugs cost money. I do not want to do wrong things to get money for drugs. I do not want to be around people who sell drugs.

7. **I want to reduce violence.** Most people who harm other people are under the influence of drugs. Drugs can make a person angry and mean. I do not want to use drugs and be angry and mean. I do not want to start fights. I do not want to harm anyone.

8. **I want to reach my goals.** I have plans for my future. Drugs can only make it hard for me to reach my goals.

9. **I want to follow school rules so I can play sports and be in school activities.** My school has drug-free rules. If I break the rules, I cannot play sports. I cannot go to school activities. I do not want to miss out.

10. **I want to get good grades.** Drugs can affect my memory. Using drugs makes it harder for me to learn. I want to do my homework and learn. I know I will have more opportunities if I get good grades.

Why Do I Need to Expect Other People to Be Drug-Free?

You must expect other people to be drug-free. Your life will be better if members of your family are drug-free. Your life will be better if your friends are drug-free.

Suppose someone you know uses drugs. This person might buy or sell drugs, too. How can this person's behavior affect you?

People who use drugs often lie about their behavior. They make up excuses for their wrong actions. They say they do not have a drug problem if asked. This is hard for someone your age. No one your age wants to have someone they know on drugs.

As a result, you might try to hide what is happening. You might lie for the person who uses drugs. You might make excuses for the person who uses drugs. You might try to clown around and show you are happy when you are not.

These actions are ways to cope with the drug use of someone you know. But they are not healthful. Inside you might feel frightened, angry, and sad. You might be confused. But these feelings are hidden. You pay a price for keeping feelings inside. When you are out of touch with anger, fear, and sadness, you are out of touch with joy. You start to feel numb. It is hard to respond to any emotions.

Get help if someone you know uses harmful drugs. Talk to a family member you trust. Suppose the family member you choose does not want to talk about it. Talk to another trusted adult. You and the person you know need help.

Expect Other People to Be Drug-Free

● No one should lie to you about his or her harmful drug use.

● No one should harm you because he or she is under the influence of drugs.

● No one should expect you to keep his or her harmful drug use a secret.

I will say NO if someone offers me a harmful drug.

How Can I Use Honest Talk with Someone Who Abuses Drugs?

Honest talk is the open sharing of feelings. Suppose a person you care about uses harmful drugs. How might you use honest talk?

- **Write down the actions you do not like.** What exactly does this person do? Suppose someone you care about drinks too much. When this person drinks, he or she yells. This person might hit you or someone else. This person might lie and say he or she has not been drinking. This person might promise to stop drinking. But the promise is not kept. These are actions you do not like.

- **Write down how you feel about the actions you do not like.** You might feel frightened. You might feel angry. You might feel sad or confused.

- **Practice saying the actions you do not like and tell how you feel about the actions.** Stand in front of a mirror. Talk out loud. "I am scared when you drink too much and yell at me." "I am confused when I see you drink and you lie about it." "I am angry that I cannot trust you because you drink too much."

- **Talk to the person who uses harmful drugs.** Use honest talk. Say the actions you do not like and tell how you feel about them. Choose a time when the person is not under the influence of drugs. Do not back down. Use good judgment. Sometimes it is best not to talk to a person who uses harmful drugs. This person might have other behaviors. For example, this person might be someone who abuses others and acts in violent ways. Do not put yourself in a position in which you might be harmed. If the person will hurt you for being honest, talk to another adult. Tell the adult what you would have said.

Keeping a Journal

You can keep what you have written in a journal. Date the entries in your journal. Then you will have a record of what has happened. This will help keep you from being in denial. You are not as likely to overlook the effects the drug abuse has on you. A journal helps in another way. You can share it with your parent, guardian, or other trusted adult. You can share it with a counselor. This can help with the treatment of the person.

How Can I Say No If I Am Pressured to Abuse Drugs?

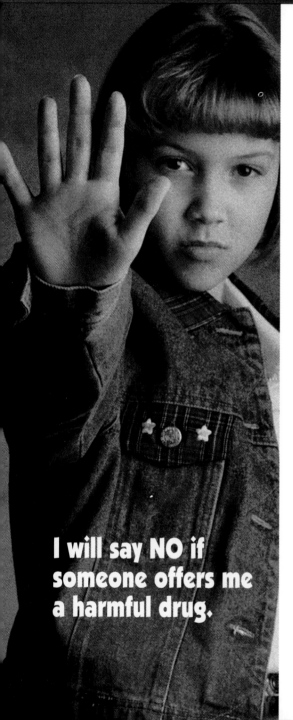

I will say NO if someone offers me a harmful drug.

Use resistance skills:

1. **Say NO in a firm voice to abusing drugs.**
   - Sound like you mean what you say.
2. **Give reasons for saying NO to using drugs.**
   - I want to obey laws.
   - I want to follow my parents' or guardian's guidelines.
   - I want to protect my safety.
   - I want to be in control of my actions.
   - I want to be a good example for others.
   - I want to reduce crime.
   - I want to reduce violence.
   - I want to reach my goals.
   - I want to follow school rules so I can play sports and be in school activities.
   - I want to get good grades.
3. **Be certain your behavior matches your words.**
   - Do not pretend to take a sip of beer from a can.
   - Do not try a drug just once.
4. **Stay away from situations in which there will be pressure to use drugs.**
   - Do not go to parties where peers will use drugs.
5. **Stay away from peers who use drugs.**
   - Choose friends who are drug-free.
6. **Tell an adult if you are pressured to use drugs.**
   - Adults can help you stick to your decision.
   - The person who pressures you needs help.
7. **Encourage your peers to be drug-free.**
   - Suggest healthful activities.

Turn Up the Volume

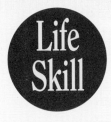

Life Skill — **I will say NO if someone offers me a harmful drug.**

Materials: Paper, pen or pencil

Directions: Suppose you say NO to drugs. Someone begins to pressure you over and over. Turn Up the Volume is a technique to make your NO firm.

Follow these four steps to make your NO firm.

1. **Say NO and give your reason.**
2. **Repeat in a firm voice. Say NO and give your reason.**
3. **Repeat in a firmer voice. Say NO and give your reason.**
4. **Walk away.**

Activity

1. **Choose one reason to be drug-free.** You can choose one reason from the list on page 181.
2. **Practice the four steps on the left.** Your teacher will call on different classmates. When he or she calls on you, stand. Then say NO and your reason. Be firmer each time and then walk away.

   NO. I want to obey laws.

   NO. I want to obey laws. (Turn up the volume.)

   NO. I want to obey laws. (Turn up the volume.)

   Walk to the back of the classroom.

Lesson 24

Review

Vocabulary

Write a separate sentence using each of the vocabulary words listed on page 180.

Health Content

Write answers to the following:

1. What are ten reasons to stay drug-free? **page 181**
2. Why should you expect others to be drug-free? **page 182**
3. How can you use honest talk with someone who abuses drugs? **page 183**
4. What are ways to say NO if you are pressured to abuse drugs? **page 184**
5. What technique can you use to make your NO firm? **page 185**

Alcohol-Free... That's Me!

Vocabulary

alcohol: a depressant drug found in some beverages.

depressant: a drug that slows down the body's functions.

blood alcohol level (BAL): the amount of alcohol in a person's blood.

alcohol-free: to say NO to using alcohol and to going to parties where there is alcohol.

alcoholism: a disease in which a person is dependent on alcohol.

recovery program: a group that supports people who are trying to change.

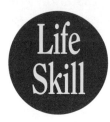

Life Skill

● **I will not drink alcohol.**

Alcohol is a depressant drug found in some beverages. Different drinks contain alcohol in different amounts. Beer and wine coolers contain 3 to 6 percent alcohol. Wine contains 12 percent alcohol. Liquor such as gin, vodka, and rum contains as much as 50 percent alcohol. Any amount of alcohol is harmful for someone your age.

The Lesson Objectives

● Discuss the depressant effects of alcohol.

● Discuss ten reasons to be alcohol-free.

● List questions you can ask to judge ads and commercials for alcohol.

● Discuss signs of alcoholism.

● Explain what happens in a recovery program.

What Are the Depressant Effects of Alcohol?

When a person drinks, alcohol passes from the stomach and small intestine into the bloodstream. Blood carries alcohol to the brain and all the body cells. Alcohol is a depressant. A **depressant** is a drug that slows down the body's functions.

How alcohol affects a person depends on a person's blood alcohol level. **Blood alcohol level (BAL)** is the amount of alcohol in a person's blood. As a person drinks more, BAL increases. The depressant effects of alcohol are greater.

Some depressant effects are present shortly after a person begins to drink. Alcohol depresses parts of the brain. The parts of the brain that control thinking are affected. A person who has been drinking does not think as clearly. A person who has been drinking might make mistakes.

The parts of the brain that control movement also are affected. A person who has been drinking will not react as quickly. The person's speech might be slurred. Bodily movements, such as walking, might be affected.

The depressant effects of alcohol can be serious. A person might get drunk or have a blackout. A person is drunk when coordination and judgment are affected. A *blackout* is a period about which a person cannot remember what happened.

Suppose a pregnant female drinks alcohol. Alcohol from her blood gets into the developing baby's blood. Alcohol depresses body functions in the developing baby. The baby is born with FAS. *Fetal* (FEE·tuhl) *alcohol syndrome* or *FAS* is birth defects in babies whose mothers drank alcohol during pregnancy. Babies born with FAS might be mentally retarded.

Alcohol Is a Toxin

Alcohol is a toxin. A toxin is a substance that is a poison. After a certain amount of alcohol is swallowed, the stomach will reject it. This is why a person might vomit after drinking.

It is against the law for some-one your age to drink or to buy alcohol.

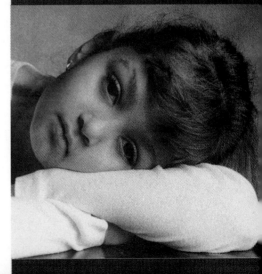

What Are Ten Reasons to Be Alcohol-Free?

To be **alcohol-free** is to say NO to using alcohol and to going to parties where there is alcohol. Suppose someone asks you why you are alcohol-free. Here are ten reasons you can give.

1. **I want to obey laws.** Drinking alcohol is illegal for people under a certain age. This age is determined by state laws. In every state, it is against the law for people your age to drink.

2. **I want to make responsible decisions.** Drinking alcohol affects reasoning and judgment. If you drink, your mind is not sharp. You are less aware of possible outcomes of decisions. You might say or do something you regret later. You could have a blackout and not remember what happened.

3. **I want my body senses to function at their best.** Drinking alcohol changes body senses. If you drink, your vision can become blurred. It is hard for you to judge distance. This is why people who have been drinking have more accidents. It also is hard to judge whether you are hot or cold.

4. **I want to keep from having accidents.** Drinking alcohol slows reaction time. Your reaction time is the length of time it takes to move after a signal. Suppose you are riding your bicycle. Someone moves into your path. You quickly brake to keep from running into the person. If you had been drinking, it would take you longer to brake. Your chances of hitting the person would be greater. People who are drinking are more likely to fall. They are more likely to drown. Some day you probably want to get a driver's license. Drinking alcohol is a leading cause of injury and death from car accidents.

Caution:
Drinking Alcohol Can Cause:

Fights	Drowning
Assault	Cirrhosis
Heart disease	Cancer
Suicide	Depression
Alcoholism	Car accidents

5. **I want to have healthful relationships.** Right now you are learning social skills. Social skills are skills that can be used to relate well with others. You might not know how to act at times. You might have a hard time talking to someone. But you learn by practicing social skills. Drinking alcohol changes how you respond to others. Drinking is a crutch. It keeps you from getting better at talking to other people.

6. **I want to get along well with my family.** Your parents or guardians do not want you to drink. If you drink, you will have to sneak to do it. You will worry about getting caught. If you get caught, your parents or guardians will be angry with you. You will have let them down. It is just not worth it to drink! Suppose you want to marry and have a family some day. Alcohol is a leading cause of divorce. Drinking alcohol during pregnancy causes fetal alcohol syndrome.

7. **I want to keep from being depressed.** Alcohol is a depressant. Suppose you are sad. If you drink, you can become more sad. Suppose you feel down because you cannot deal with problems. If you drink, it is even harder to deal with problems. You think your problems are worse. Most young people who make a suicide attempt had been drinking.

8. **I want to stay away from fights.** Suppose you are very angry. If you drink, you become more angry. The reasoning part of your brain does not work as well. You do not manage anger well. You are more likely to get into fights.

9. **I want to protect myself from diseases such as heart disease, cancer, and liver disease.** If you drink, alcohol enters your blood. Your blood carries the alcohol to all of your body organs. Alcohol weakens the heart muscles. It can cause the heart to have fat around it. It can cause you to have an irregular heartbeat. Alcohol can change cells. Drinking raises the risk of several cancers. These cancers are the mouth, throat, esophagus, pancreas, and liver. Females who drink have a greater chance of breast cancer. Drinking causes other changes in the liver. The liver gets larger and becomes fatty. *Cirrhosis* (suh·ROH·suhs) is a disease in which liver cells are damaged.

10. **I do not want to have alcoholism.** **Alcoholism** is a disease in which a person is dependent on alcohol. This disease runs in families. Suppose someone in your family has alcoholism. There might be something in your family's biological makeup. You might be at higher risk than other people for having this disease. There is only one way to keep from having alcoholism—do not drink.

What Beer Commercials Do Not Tell You

Activity

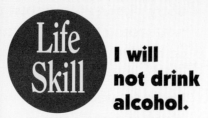

Life Skill I will not drink alcohol.

Materials: Television time with your parent or guardian, paper, pen or pencil, magazine ad for beer

Directions: This activity helps you understand the messages that are in beer commercials. It teaches you to respond to these messages in healthful ways.

1. **Learn about media literacy.** Here are facts to help you. Media literacy is being able to see and evaluate the messages you get from media. Some examples of media are television, radio, magazines, newspapers, books, and the Internet. You need to have media literacy:

   • to understand messages in the media.

   • to understand the appeals in messages that are intended to influence you.

   • to respond to messages in media in a responsible way.

2. **Ask your parent or guardian to watch a beer commercial with you.** If this is not possible, ask if it is OK for you to watch a beer commercial on your own. (If TV is not available, check out a magazine ad for beer.)

3. **Answer the following questions.**

   • Who wrote the commercial?

   • How do you know the beer commercial is for young adults?

   • What is the beer commercial trying to get young adults to do?

   • Is the beer commercial trying to get young adults to do something responsible? (Think about the *Guidelines for Making Responsible Decisions™.*)

   • Did the beer commercial leave out any facts? Why?

4. **List five facts you know about alcohol that were not in the beer commercial.**

5. **Share your answers and your five facts with classmates.**

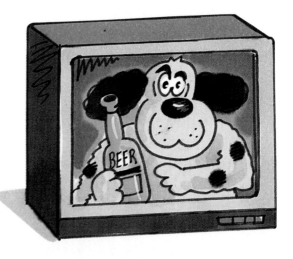

What Are Signs That a Person Has Alcoholism?

Alcoholism (AL·kuh·HAW·LI·zuhm) is a disease in which a person is dependent on alcohol. The signs of this disease are not the same in all people who have it. Some people who have alcoholism appear drunk often. But this does not describe other people who have alcoholism. You cannot point out these people when you pass them on the street. You would need to know more about them before you could tell they had this disease.

People who have alcoholism have one or more of the following signs. They might,

- have problems caused by their drinking.
- refuse to say that drinking is a problem for them.
- lie about their drinking or try to hide it.
- have blackouts.
- have a change in personality caused by drinking.

Suppose someone you know has alcoholism. Perhaps the person is a close friend. Talk to the person when he or she is not drinking. Use honest talk. Tell the person the actions you do not like. Explain how you feel about these actions. Encourage the person to get help.

In many cases, the person will say he or she does not have a problem. The person might even try to blame you in some way. These are signs of alcoholism. **You are not at fault. There is nothing wrong with you. You cannot get someone to stop drinking who does not want to stop.**

Talk to your parent, guardian, or other trusted adult. An adult can get the person the help that is needed. People who have alcoholism need two kinds of treatment. They need treatment for the physical effects of the disease. They need treatment for the emotional effects of the disease.

Alcoholism Is a Leading Cause of Premature Death

The disease alcoholism ranks as a leading cause of premature death. Premature death is death before the expected time. Alcoholism helps brings on other causes of death. These include:

- Accidents
- Homicide
- Suicide
- Heart disease
- Cancer
- Cirrhosis

What Do People Do in a Recovery Program?

A **recovery program** is a group that supports people who are trying to change. There are many kinds of recovery programs. It is not a sign of weakness to join one. It is a way of getting others to help out when it is hard to change.

People who have alcoholism have a hard disease to treat. They can get medical help to treat health problems. But they might go back to drinking if other parts of their lives do not change. They have depended on drinking for emotional reasons. This means they must learn new ways to deal with feelings.

This is where recovery programs help. *Alcoholics Anonymous (AA)* is a recovery program for people who have alcoholism. Other people who have alcoholism are in their group. They share hard times with each other. They encourage each other to try new ways of coping. Suppose a member of the group wants to drink. This member can call another person in AA. This person talks to the person. They help each other keep the promise not to drink.

There are recovery programs for other people, too. *Al-Anon* is a recovery program for people who are close to someone who has an addiction. Family members and friends join Al-Anon. *Alateen* is a recovery program for teens who are close to someone who has an addiction.

Suppose someone your age goes to Al-Anon or Alateen. What do young people do in these groups? They share the tough times they have been through. They share their feelings. They help each other set limits. They will expect people close to them to be drug-free. They will expect to be treated with respect.

Alcoholism: The Family Link

Suppose one or both of your biological parents has alcoholism. Suppose one or more of your biological grandparents has alcoholism. Then you are at risk for having this disease. But even if this is so, you never have to have alcoholism. Pledge not to drink alcohol.

Use...
Guidelines for Making Responsible Decisions™

A classmate invites you over after school. When you get there, his parents are not home. He offers you a wine cooler. He says it is like drinking fruit juice.

Use a separate sheet of paper. Answer "yes" or "no" to each of the following questions. Explain each answer.

1. Is it healthful for you to drink a wine cooler?
2. Is it safe for you to drink a wine cooler?
3. Do you follow rules and laws if you drink a wine cooler?
4. Do you show respect for yourself and others if you drink a wine cooler?
5. Do you follow your family's guidelines if you drink a wine cooler?
6. Do you show good character if you drink a wine cooler?

What is the responsible decision to make?

Lesson 25

Review

Vocabulary

Write a separate sentence using each of the vocabulary words listed on page 186.

Health Content
Write answers to the following:

1. What are the depressant effects of alcohol? **page 187**
2. What are ten reasons to be alcohol-free? **pages 188–189**
3. What are five questions to ask when you see an ad or commercial for alcohol? **page 190**
4. What are signs of alcoholism? **page 191**
5. What do people do in a recovery program? **page 192**

Tobacco-Free... That's Me!

Vocabulary

tobacco-free: to say NO to using tobacco and to breathing smoke from tobacco products.

nicotine: a stimulant drug found in tobacco.

secondhand smoke: exhaled smoke and sidestream smoke.

sidestream smoke: smoke from a burning cigarette or cigar.

carcinogen: a substance that causes cancer.

smokeless tobacco: tobacco that is chewed.

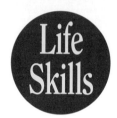

Life Skills

- I will not use tobacco.
- I will protect myself from secondhand smoke.

Tobacco is a plant that contains nicotine. Tobacco products include cigarettes, cigars, and smokeless tobacco. Most young people today are tobacco-free. To be **tobacco-free** is to say NO to using tobacco and to breathing smoke from tobacco products. Protect your health. Make the decision to be tobacco-free and stick to it.

The Lesson Objectives

- Tell why you can get addicted if you try tobacco.
- Discuss reasons not to smoke now or later.
- Discuss reasons to stay away from second-hand smoke.
- Discuss reasons not to use smokeless tobacco.
- List questions you can use to judge ads for tobacco products.

Why Could I Get Addicted If I Try Tobacco?

Tobacco products—cigarettes, cigars, snuff—all have nicotine in them. **Nicotine** (NI·kuh·TEEN) is a stimulant drug found in tobacco. As a stimulant, nicotine speeds up body functions. It speeds up the heart rate. It increases blood pressure. It speeds up the number of times you breathe each minute.

Nicotine has other effects. It stimulates the brain. It provides a "pick-me-up" feeling. This feeling happens right after using it. Suppose someone smokes a cigarette. This person gets this feeling right away. But this feeling does not last. If the person likes the feeling, he or she will want to smoke another cigarette right away. This is how people get addicted.

You can get addicted to nicotine if you use tobacco just once. Its effects on the brain are that strong. Then it is really hard to give it up. You probably have known someone who tried to quit smoking. The person might have been very cranky. The person probably had headaches and felt nervous.

Many people who try to stop using tobacco go right back. This is why it is best not to ever take a puff of a cigarette. It is best not to chew smokeless tobacco even once.

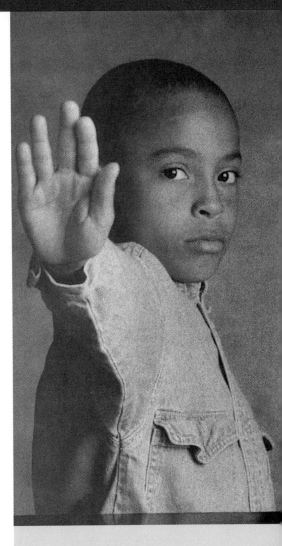

The Truth About Tobacco Products

- Tobacco products contain nicotine.
- Nicotine causes addiction.
- A person can become addicted to nicotine the first time he or she uses tobacco.

What Are Ten Reasons Not to Smoke Cigarettes and Cigars?

Suppose someone asks you why you do not smoke cigarettes or cigars. Here are reasons you can give.

1. **I want to obey my parents or guardian.** The use of tobacco products is harmful. Your parents or guardian want you to protect your health. They do not want you to begin a harmful habit. They know how hard it is to break the habit if you start. Suppose one of your parents or your guardian has smoked or smokes now. They know how hard it is to quit.

2. **I do not want to get addicted to nicotine.** Would you accept a dare to run in front of a moving car just once? Suppose a friend says you could probably make it. You would be a fool to take the dare. The possible harm is too great. Nicotine is a powerful drug. It is just as addictive as cocaine and heroin. It is too risky to try such a dangerous drug.

3. **I want to protect my heart and blood vessels.** Nicotine speeds up your heart beat. It increases your blood pressure. Your heart and blood vessels get extra wear and tear on them. You might not think this is a big deal. You are unlikely to have a heart attack or stroke at this point. But harmful changes can occur in your blood vessels now.

4. **I want to have cardiorespiratory endurance for sports.** There is carbon monoxide in smoke from cigarettes and cigars. Carbon monoxide (KAR·buhn muh·NAHK·SYD) is an odorless, colorless, and poisonous gas. This gas gets into the blood if you smoke. Your heart beats more often to get oxygen to cells. The result—you get out of breath sooner if you smoke.

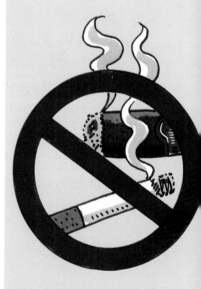

5. **I do not want respiratory infections.** If you smoke, cilia do not work as they should. Cilia (SI·lee·uh) are tiny hairs that line the air passages. Cilia keep germs and pollutants from getting into your lungs. If you smoke, the cilia stop working. It is easier to get colds and flu. You can get other diseases. Emphysema (EMP·fuh·ZEE·muh) is a disease in which air sacs in the lungs are damaged. Asthma is a chronic condition in which it is hard to breathe.

6. **I want to protect myself from cancer now and later.** Smoking causes more than 30 percent of all cancer deaths. Smoking causes most lung cancer deaths. It raises the risk of other cancers like liver, kidney, stomach, and breast. Suppose you smoke and quit. You have less risk of cancer than if you kept smoking. However, here is a fact to know. If you smoke at all, you increase your chance of cancer for the rest of your life! This is why you cannot try smoking—even once.

7. **I want to keep the air clean for other people to breathe.** If you smoke, other people breathe the smoke. Keep the air free of smoke for others.

8. **I want to be safe from fires and accidents.** If you smoke, you might forget where you put the lighted cigarette or cigar. It can cause fire. Burning ashes can drop on your clothes and burn them. It is hard to watch what you are doing and hold a cigar or cigarette. People who are smoking have more accidents.

9. **I want to be well-groomed.** You have self-respect when you try to look your best. Other people notice how you look. If you smoke, they see a cloud of smoke by you. Your clothes will smell. Your teeth will be stained. Your breath will smell.

10. **I want to spend money wisely.** Never waste money—not even a penny. If you have money to smoke, you have money to save. Save your money for the future.

Cigar Smoking

The American Lung Association wants you to know that cigar smoking is dangerous. They provide a fact sheet on cigar smoking. Consider these facts. Suppose you compare cigar smokers to non-smokers. Cigar smokers are four to ten times more likely to get cancer of the larynx, esophagus, and mouth. This risk is greater if cigar smokers drink. The practice of holding an unlit cigar in the mouth is harmful, too. The nicotine in an unlit cigar can get into the bloodstream. Breathing cigar smoke is risky too. You breathe in over 4,000 chemicals—23 are poisons and 43 cause cancer.

What Are Five Reasons to Stay Away from Secondhand Smoke?

Secondhand smoke is exhaled smoke and sidestream smoke. **Sidestream smoke** is smoke from a burning cigarette or cigar. Suppose someone asks you why you ask people not to smoke. They ask you why you sit in nonsmoking sections of restaurants. They ask you why you support laws to stop smoking in public places. Here are reasons you can give.

1. **I have learned that breathing secondhand smoke causes the same health problems as smoking does.** Suppose you are in a room for one hour with people who are smoking. Breathing this smoke is as harmful as smoking 25 cigarettes with filters.

2. **I do not want to irritate my eyes, throat, and lungs.** If you are around smoke, your eyes might sting. You might cough. You do not get as much oxygen with each breath you take. You get out of breath sooner.

3. **I do not want my hair and clothes to smell.** Cigarette and cigar smoke have an unpleasant odor. Smoke stays in clothes. Your clothes smell even after you leave a place where people have been smoking. Some people might smell the smoke on you. They might think you smoke even though you do not.

4. **I want to protect myself against heart disease and cancer.** Secondhand smoke is a carcinogen. A **carcinogen** (kar·SI·nuh·juhn) is a substance that causes cancer. Secondhand smoke is a leading cause of heart disease. People who live with a person who smokes have a much greater chance of having heart disease.

5. **I want to protect myself against asthma and respiratory diseases.** Breathing secondhand smoke raises the risk of asthma. It raises the risk of chronic bronchitis, too.

Use Honest Talk If Someone Lights Up a Cigarette or Cigar
- **State the actions that concern you.**
"I do not want you to smoke around me."

- **Tell the effect these actions have on you.**
"I cough and sneeze when I breathe smoke."

What Are Five Reasons Not to Use Smokeless Tobacco?

Smokeless tobacco is tobacco that is chewed. Smokeless tobacco is very harmful. If you try it, you can get some of the harmful effects right away. For example, it can cause oral cancer in young people. Suppose someone asks you why you do not use smokeless tobacco. Here are reasons you can give.

1. **I do not want to be addicted to nicotine.**
   Smokeless tobacco contains nicotine. Nicotine is a powerful drug. It is just as addictive as crack, cocaine, and heroin. It is too risky to try such a dangerous drug.

2. **I want to protect my heart and blood vessels.**
   Nicotine speeds up your heart beat. It increases your blood pressure. Your heart and blood vessels get extra wear and tear. You might not think this is a big deal. You are unlikely to have a heart attack or stroke at this point. But harmful changes can occur in your blood vessels now.

3. **I want to protect myself from cancer.** Suppose you used smokeless tobacco. The tobacco mixes with your saliva to form tobacco juice. This juice has carcinogens in it. It changes the cells in your teeth and gums. White spots can appear. These white spots can become cancer.

4. **I want to protect my teeth and gums.** Tobacco juice causes gingivitis. Your gums become sore and bleed easily. It causes periodontal disease. The gums pull away from your teeth. Teeth become loose and can fall out.

5. **I want to protect my mouth and stomach.**
   Tobacco juice can cause ulcers. An ulcer is an open sore. You can get ulcers in your mouth and stomach.

Your parents or guardian do not want you to use smokeless tobacco. They do not want you to get addicted to nicotine.

Most athletes such as baseball players do not use chewing tobacco. They know chewing tobacco is harmful. They do not want to get cancer or have their teeth fall out.

What Cigarette Ads Should Say

Activity

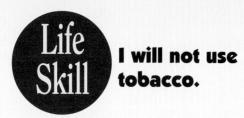

Life Skill I will not use tobacco.

Materials: Magazine ad for cigarettes, paper, pen or pencil, computer (optional)

Directions: This activity helps you understand the messages in cigarette ads. It teaches you to respond in a healthful way.

Surgeon General's Warning:
Cigarette Smoke Contains Carbon Monoxide.

Surgeon General's Warning:
Quitting Smoking Now Greatly Reduces Serious Risks to Your Health.

Surgeon General's Warning:
Smoking Causes Lung Cancer, Heart Disease, Emphysema, and May Complicate Pregnancy.

Surgeon General's Warning:
Smoking by Pregnant Women May Result in Fetal Injury, Premature Births, and Low Birth Weights.

1. **Learn about media literacy.** Here are facts to help you. Media literacy is being able to see and evaluate the messages you get from media. Some examples of media are television, radio, magazines, newspapers, books, and the Internet. You need to have media literacy:
   - to understand messages in the media.
   - to understand the appeals in messages that are intended to influence you.
   - to respond to media messages in a responsible way.

2. **Evaluate the magazine ad for cigarettes.** Answer the following questions.
   - Who wrote the ad?
   - How do you know the ad tries to convince young people?
   - What does the ad try to get young people to do?
   - Is the magazine ad trying to get young people to do something responsible? (Think about the *Guidelines for Making Responsible Decisions™.*)
   - Did the magazine ad leave out any facts? Why?

3. **Make your own magazine ad.** Create an ad that shows what people should know about smoking. Use one of the warnings from the Surgeon General.

Where Can People Get Help to Quit Using Tobacco?

A *tobacco cessation* (se·SAY·shuhn) *program* is a program to quit tobacco use. There are programs that help people stop smoking. There are programs that help people stop using smokeless tobacco. These are places where people can find out about these programs.

- The local chapter of the American Cancer Society (ACS)
- The local chapter of the American Heart Association (AHA)
- The local chapter of the American Lung Association (ALA)
- Your school
- The health department in your community
- Community providers, such as hospitals

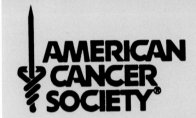

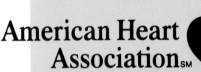
Fighting Heart Disease and Stroke

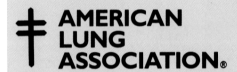

Lesson 26

Review

Vocabulary

Write a separate sentence using each of the vocabulary words listed on page 194.

Health Content

Write answers to the following:

1. Why can you get addicted if you try tobacco? **page 195**

2. What are ten reasons not to smoke? **pages 196–197**

3. What are five reasons to stay away from second-hand smoke? **page 198**

4. What are five reasons not to use smokeless tobacco? **page 199**

5. What are five questions to ask when you see an ad for cigarettes? **page 200**

Illegal Drug Use?... NO WAY!

Vocabulary

stimulant: a drug that speeds up body functions.

depressant: a drug that slows down body functions.

narcotic: a drug that slows down the nervous system and relieves pain.

inhalant: a chemical that is breathed.

marijuana: an illegal drug that affects mood and short-term memory.

steroids: drugs that act like hormones.

hallucinogens: illegal drugs that cause hallucinations.

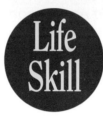 **Life Skill**

• **I will not be involved in illegal drug use.**

Some drugs are against the law to buy, sell, or use. Some drugs are against the law to buy, sell, or use without a prescription. *Illegal drug use* is using illegal drugs or using legal drugs in a way that breaks the law. There are stiff punishments for illegal drug use.

The Lesson Objectives

● Discuss the effects of stimulants.

● Discuss the effects of depressants.

● Discuss the effects of narcotics.

● Discuss the effects of inhalants.

● Discuss the effects of marijuana.

● Discuss the effects of anabolic steroids.

● Discuss the effects of hallucinogens.

What Are the Effects of Stimulants?

A **stimulant** (STIM·yuh·luhnt) is a drug that speeds up body functions.

Caffeine use can cause addiction. *Caffeine* is a stimulant found in chocolate, coffee, tea, some soda pops, and some drugs. Caffeine produces a "pick-me-up" feeling. But caffeine also irritates your stomach. It can give you headaches and make your heart beat fast. You can get addicted to caffeine. It is best to limit or not have caffeine.

Nicotine use can cause addiction. *Nicotine* is a stimulant drug found in tobacco. Nicotine is in cigarettes, cigars, and smokeless tobacco. A person who holds an unlit cigar in the mouth gets nicotine in the body. You already have learned about this drug. You can get addicted to nicotine right away. It is best never to try tobacco.

Cocaine and crack use is illegal. *Cocaine* is an illegal stimulant made from coca bush leaves. *Crack* is an illegal stimulant that is stronger than cocaine. These drugs cause addiction. At first, a person gets a high. Then the person becomes very depressed. Some users make suicide attempts. Some users overdose. Users who share needles to inject cocaine or crack might become infected with HIV. HIV is the pathogen that destroys helper T cells and causes AIDS.

Amphetamine use is illegal without a prescription. An *amphetamine* (am·FE·tuh·MEEN) is a stimulant drug used to treat sleep disorders and attention problems. These drugs are addictive. Users can lose interest in daily activities.

Stimulants

- Speed up the heart rate
- Speed up blood pressure
- Keep users awake
- Make users restless and cranky
- Cause loss of appetite
- Cause blurred vision
- Produce tolerance
- Can be addictive
- Can cause death by heart or breathing failure

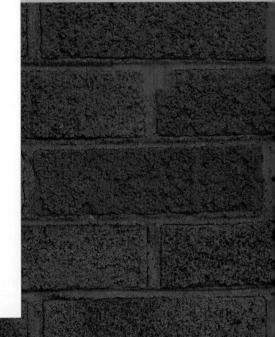

What Are the Effects of Depressants?

A **depressant** is a drug that slows down body functions.

Alcohol use is illegal for someone your age. Alcohol is a drug found in some beverages. It is in liquor, beer, wine, and wine coolers. Alcohol is a depressant. It is illegal for you to buy or drink alcohol. The effects of alcohol are greater in a person your age. Suppose someone your age drinks alcohol and uses another depressant drug. This can cause overdose. An overdose is an excessive amount. This is very dangerous.

Tranquilizer use is illegal without a prescription. A *tranquilizer* (TRAN·kwuh·LY·zuhr) is a drug that relieves anxiety. A doctor might prescribe this kind of drug for some people. Users must follow directions. These drugs can be addictive. They slow reaction time. Users cannot do things like mow grass or drive a car. They might have an accident. Users might get dizzy or have headaches. Taking this drug with alcohol can cause death.

Barbiturate use is illegal without a prescription. A *barbiturate* (bar·BI·chuh·ruht) is a drug that relieves anxiety and causes sleepiness. A doctor might prescribe this kind of drug for some people. Users must follow directions. These drugs can be addictive. They make users very sleepy. Users cannot do things that need fast action. They might have an accident. Taking this drug with alcohol can cause death.

Depressants

- Slow the heart rate
- Reduce blood pressure
- Cause sleepiness
- Relax muscles
- Produce drunken-like behavior
- Reduce pain
- Slow down the thinking part of the brain
- Can produce coma
- Can be addictive
- Can cause death if used while drinking alcohol

I will not be involved in illegal drug use.

What Are the Effects of Narcotics?

A **narcotic** (nar·KAH·tik) is a drug that slows down the nervous system and relieves pain.

Morphine use is illegal without a prescription.
Morphine (MOR·feen) is a narcotic used to control pain. A doctor might prescribe morphine for someone who has a late stage of cancer. Their pain is difficult to bear without this drug.

Codeine use is illegal without a prescription. *Codeine* (KOH·deen) is a narcotic painkiller made from morphine. A doctor might prescribe a cough syrup with codeine in it. Users take it to keep from coughing over and over. A doctor might prescribe it for someone after surgery. A dentist might prescribe it for someone who has had dental work. Users take it to relieve pain. It is risky to drink and take codeine. Some users have side effects. They get dizzy and sick to their stomach. They get very bad headaches.

Heroin use is illegal. *Heroin* (HEHR·uh·wuhn) is an illegal narcotic made from morphine. There is no medical use for heroin. Users who share a needle to inject heroin might become infected with HIV. HIV is the pathogen that destroys helper T cells and causes AIDS.

Narcotics

- Slow heart rate
- Slow breathing rate
- Relieve pain
- Cause nausea
- Produce sleepiness
- Can be addictive
- Can cause breathing to stop
- Can cause death if used while drinking alcohol

I will not be involved in illegal drug use.

What Are the Effects of Inhalants?

An **inhalant** (in·HAY·luhnt) is a chemical that is breathed. There are chemicals in household cleaning products. There are chemicals in glue, nail polish, shoe polish, and hair spray. Always get fresh air when you use these products.

Inhalants

- Slow down the nervous system
- Damage the lungs, throat, nose, and mouth
- Cause users to have seizures
- Kill brain cells
- Change mood and behavior
- Cause different kinds of cancer
- Can cause sudden death

Fume Watch

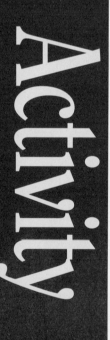

Activity

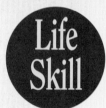

Life Skill **I will not be involved in illegal drug use.**

Materials: Paper, pen or pencil

Directions:
Pretend you own a company. Your company produces a product that has chemicals in it. You want people to be safe when using your product.

1. **Choose a product whose fumes might be harmful.** You might select glue, a household cleaner, nail polish, nail polish remover, shoe polish, or hair spray.
2. **Write a label to warn users about the fumes.** Tell users to get fresh air when the product is used. Tell the harmful effects of inhaling fumes.
3. **Put your label on a bulletin board.**

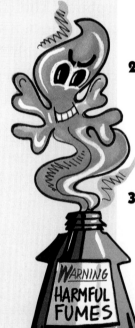

WARNING HARMFUL FUMES

What Are the Effects of Marijuana?

Marijuana (MEHR·uh·WAH·nuh) is an illegal drug that affects mood and short-term memory. *Hashish* (ha·SHEESH) is a drug made from marijuana that has stronger effects. The main ingredient in these drugs is THC. THC changes the way a user thinks and feels. Marijuana has more tar in it than do cigarettes. This puts users at risk for respiratory diseases and cancer.

Marijuana

- Speeds up heart rate
- Increases appetite
- Causes red eyes and dry mouth
- Changes mood
- Causes short-term memory loss
- Slows reaction time
- Affects the users performance in school
- Can cause users to panic
- Can cause lung cancer
- Can cause asthma attacks
- Can cause emotional dependence

Use... Guidelines for Making Responsible Decisions™

A classmate pressures you to eat a brownie with marijuana in it. She says it is not harmful if you do not smoke it.

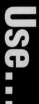

Use a separate sheet of paper. Answer "yes" or "no" to each of the following questions. Explain each answer.

1. Is it healthful for you to eat a marijuana brownie?
2. Is it safe for you to eat a marijuana brownie?
3. Do you follow rules and laws if you eat a marijuana brownie?
4. Do you show respect for yourself and others if you eat a marijuana brownie?
5. Do you follow your family's guidelines if you eat a marijuana brownie?
6. Do you show good character if you eat a marijuana brownie?

What is the responsible decision to make?

What Are the Effects of Steroids?

Steroids (STEHR·oydz) are drugs that act like hormones. There are legal and illegal uses for these drugs. Suppose someone has a respiratory infection. It goes into the lungs. The person has difficulty breathing. A doctor might prescribe one kind of steroid. This kind reduces the inflammation in the lungs.

Suppose someone has an injury from playing sports. The person might have tennis elbow. There is swelling around the elbow. A doctor might prescribe a steroid to reduce the swelling. It might be injected into the body. These uses of steroids are legal.

Anabolic steroids are drugs that act like the male hormone, testosterone. A doctor must prescribe these drugs. They are injected or taken by mouth. There are some medical uses. Some young people take these drugs without a prescription. They take them for wrong reasons. They take them to get bigger and stronger muscles. Use of steroids in this way is risky.

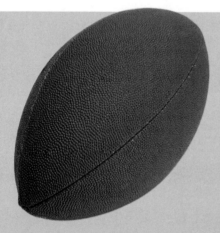

Use of anabolic steroids for sports is banned. Their use harms health. Their use does not allow for fair competition.

Anabolic steroids

- Cause acne
- Cause yellow skin and eyes
- Cause tiredness
- Cause muscle cramps
- Cause headaches
- Can cause males to have larger breasts
- Can harm reproductive organs
- Can cause females to have smaller breasts
- Can cause a female to get a deep voice
- Can cause a female to grow body hair
- Can cause heart attack and stroke
- Can cause kidney failure
- Can cause liver cancer
- Can make users mean
- Can cause depression

What Are the Effects of Hallucinogens?

Hallucinogens (huh·LOO·suhn·uh·juhnz) are illegal drugs that cause hallucinations. A *hallucination* is something that is seen or heard that is not real.

LSD use is illegal. *LSD* is an illegal hallucinogen that causes flashbacks. A flashback is seeing or hearing something that is not real long after taking a drug. Flashbacks can be scary. LSD can stay in the body a long time. Users can have poor school performance.

PCP use is illegal. *PCP* is an illegal hallucinogen that speeds up and slows down the body. Users get very mean. They might start fights and harm other people. PCP use can cause death.

Hallucinogens

- Cause users to see and hear things that are not real
- Change a person's sense of time and distance
- Cause strange behavior
- Can cause users to shake
- Cause tolerance
- Cause emotional dependence
- Produce effects that last several hours

Lesson 27

Review

Vocabulary

Write a separate sentence using each of the vocabulary words listed on page 202.

Health Content

Write answers to the following:

1. What are the effects of stimulants? Depressants? **pages 203–204**
2. What are the effects of narcotics? Inhalants? **pages 205–206**
3. What are the effects of marijuana? **page 207**
4. What are the effects of anabolic steroids? **page 208**
5. What are the effects of hallucinogens? **page 209**

Unit 6 Review

Health Content

Review your answers for each Lesson Review in this unit. Write answers to the following questions.

1. Why should OTC drugs be kept in their original containers? **Lesson 23 page 175**

2. How does drug misuse differ from drug abuse? **Lesson 23 page 176**

3. What might you do if someone you know uses harmful drugs? **Lesson 24 page 182**

4. What are ten reasons to say NO to harmful drug use? **Lesson 24 page 184**

5. What causes fetal alcohol syndrome? **Lesson 25 page 187**

6. How does drinking affect the heart? **Lesson 25 page 189**

7. How does smoking affect cardiorespiratory endurance? **Lesson 26 page 196**

8. What percentage of cancer deaths are caused by smoking? **Lesson 26 page 197**

9. What foods and beverages contain caffelne? **Lesson 27 page 203**

10. How can sniffing glue harm health? **Lesson 27 page 206**

Guidelines for Making Responsible Decisions™

Some classmates want to play a drinking game. They try to flip quarters to hit a beer can. The person who comes closest to hitting the can chooses someone to chug a beer. They want you to play. Use a separate sheet of paper. Answer "yes" or "no" to each of the following questions. Explain each answer.

1. Is it healthful to play drinking games?
2. Is it safe to play drinking games?
3. Do you follow rules and laws if you play drinking games?
4. Do you show respect for yourself and others if you play drinking games?
5. Do you follow your family's guidelines if you play drinking games?
6. Do you show good character if you play drinking games?

What is the responsible decision to make?

Family Involvement

Ask your parents or guardian what to do in the following situation. You are at a party or someone's home. Your peers want you to try drugs. Discuss how to contact them. Discuss how to leave the situation in a safe way.

Vocabulary

Number a sheet of paper from 1–10. Read each definition. Next to each number on your sheet of paper, write the vocabulary word that matches the definition.

illegal drug use	carcinogen
nicotine	addiction
blackout	marijuana
drug-free	honest talk
alcohol	over-the-counter (OTC) drug

1. To say NO to all harmful drug use. **Lesson 24**

2. A medicine that you can buy without a doctor's order. **Lesson 23**

3. A depressant drug found in some beverages. **Lesson 25**

4. A period in which a person cannot remember what happened. **Lesson 25**

5. Sharing your feelings about actions that upset you. **Lesson 24**

6. A stimulant found in tobacco. **Lesson 26**

7. A strong desire to do something even though it is harmful. **Lesson 23**

8. A substance that causes cancer. **Lesson 26**

9. Using illegal drugs or using legal drugs in a way that breaks the law. **Lesson 27**

10. An illegal drug that affects mood and short-term memory. **Lesson 27**

Health Literacy

Effective Communication

A classmate is on the soccer team with you. She has cigarettes in her book bag. If she smokes, she will get kicked off the team. On a sheet of paper, write honest talk you might use with her.

Self-Directed Learning

Write a two-page report on a disease that is caused by smoking. Include a bibliography with three references.

Critical Thinking

Answer the following question on a sheet of paper. Why should a baby's parent or guardian keep the baby away from cigarette smoke?

Responsible Citizenship

Draw a poster for a restaurant. The poster should tell reasons to sit in the nonsmoking section.

Multicultural Health

Find a magazine from a different country. Look for a cigarette ad. Compare the ad to a cigarette ad from your country. How are they the same? How are they different?

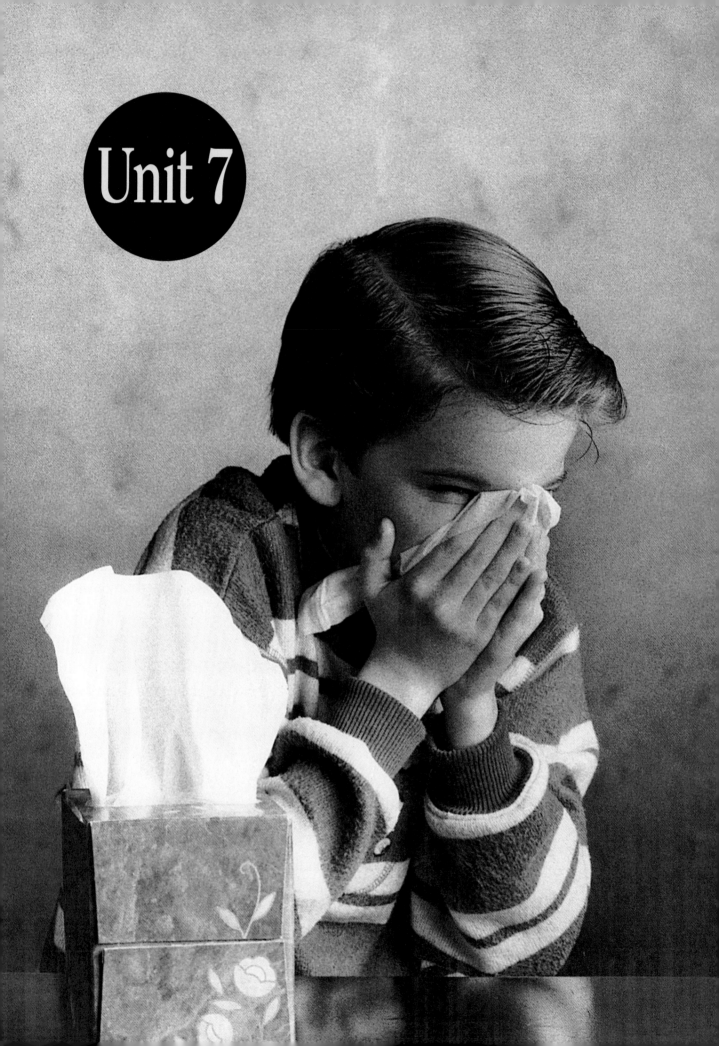

Unit 7

Communicable and Chronic Diseases

Stop the Spread of Pathogens

Vocabulary

pathogen: a germ that causes disease.

bacteria: one-celled living things.

virus: a pathogen that makes copies of itself.

antibody: a substance in the blood that helps fight pathogens.

immune: to be protected from a certain disease.

vaccine: a medicine that has dead or weak pathogens in it.

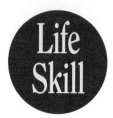

Life Skill

● **I will choose habits that prevent the spread of germs.**

Suppose someone next to you is sneezing and coughing. This person might have a cold. How can you keep from getting it? When you have a cold, what can you do to keep from spreading it to someone else? You need to know what causes diseases and what can be done to prevent them. You need to know how not to spread diseases to other people.

The Lesson Objectives

● Discuss the different kinds of pathogens.

● Explain ways that pathogens are spread.

● Describe how body defenses protect you.

What Are Different Kinds of Pathogens?

A **pathogen** (PA·thuh·juhn) is a germ that causes disease. There are five different kinds of pathogens.

One type of pathogen is bacteria. **Bacteria** (bak·TEER·ee·uh) are one-celled living things. They are too small to be seen without a microscope. There are many kinds of bacteria. Most are helpful, but some cause disease. Harmful bacteria can enter the body and multiply. They can cause illness. Strep throat, ear infections, and some pneumonias are caused by bacteria. Antibiotics (an·ty·by·AH·tiks) are medicines that can kill bacteria.

A **virus** (VY·ruhs) is a pathogen that makes copies of itself. Viruses can only be seen with a special microscope. Viruses attack body cells. When a virus enters a cell, it causes the cell to make more viruses. When the viruses multiply, they cause a person to become ill. The common cold, the flu, and measles are illnesses caused by viruses.

Another kind of pathogen is a fungus. A *fungus* (FUHN·guhs) is a plant-like living thing. Some types of fungus are helpful, but some can cause disease. Athlete's foot, ringworm, and nail infections are examples of diseases caused by different kinds of fungi.

Rickettsia (ri·KET·see·uh) are pathogens that grow inside living cells and resemble bacteria. They are smaller than bacteria. Rocky Mountain spotted fever and typhus are two diseases caused by rickettsia.

Protozoa (proh·tuh·ZOH·uh) are tiny, single-celled animals. Malaria and African sleeping sickness are diseases caused by protozoa.

Guess the Pathogen

How do doctors know what pathogen you have? They take a sample of mucus in your nose or throat, a skin scraping, or a sample of blood. They send it to a lab. Medical technologists work in laboratories. They might grow bacteria and fungi (FUN·gy) on a plate called a petri (PEE·tree) dish. They might grow viruses in a test tube. They might use special tests to find antibodies to a certain pathogen in your blood. The doctor treats your illness when he or she knows what pathogen you have.

How Are Pathogens Spread?

Pathogens, or germs, are spread in five different ways.

Pathogens are spread by touching contaminated objects. Contaminated means the object has pathogens on it. Suppose your friend has a cold and sneezes into his hand. He touches a doorknob. Other people who touch the doorknob get the pathogens on their hand. If they touch their noses, mouths, or eyes, those germs can enter their bodies.

Pathogens are spread by breathing air that contains pathogens. A person who sneezes or coughs can spread pathogens into the air. Another person who breathes this air will breathe in pathogens. These pathogens can enter the lungs and make the person ill.

Pathogens can be spread by eating foods contaminated by insects. If a person eats foods that flies or other insects have touched, that person can become ill. Insects can become contaminated with pathogens when crawling on trash or garbage. When they move to food, they spread their pathogens. People who eat that food can become ill.

Pathogens can be spread by eating contaminated food. Some meat and chicken might contain pathogens. If the meat and chicken are not cooked thoroughly, the pathogens might not be killed. When the food is eaten, the pathogens enter the body and might cause illness.

A person can become ill by eating foods that have not been properly handled or stored. It is important for people who prepare or serve food to follow safe food handling procedures.

You learned about safe food handling procedures in Lesson 16. Always wash your hands with soap and water before preparing food. The pathogens on your hands can get into the food. You should not prepare food if you have cuts or sores on your hands.

Pathogens can be spread by drinking contaminated water. If you drink water that contains pathogens, you can become ill. Water can become contaminated by wastes that have been dumped into water sources. If a water pipe breaks or leaks, pathogens can get into the water system. The water system will be contaminated. If this water is not properly treated, the water will be unsafe to use. Water can be treated by boiling or using certain chemicals. Do not cook, bathe, or drink untreated water. Do not swim in a lake with polluted water. Pathogens can enter your body if you swallow the water.

Pathogens can be spread through animal bites. Pathogens can enter the body through breaks in the skin. If a dog or cat bites or scratches you, pathogens can enter your body. Some mosquitoes, ticks, and fleas carry pathogens.

Ways to Prevent the Spread of Pathogens

You can prevent the spread of pathogens by keeping away from anyone who has an illness that can be spread. If someone is ill, try not to get near this person. Try not to touch anything this person has touched. Keep away from others when you are ill to prevent infecting them. Wash your hands after using the restroom and before eating. Wash your hands when you are around someone who is sick. Keep your hands away from your eyes, mouth, and nose.

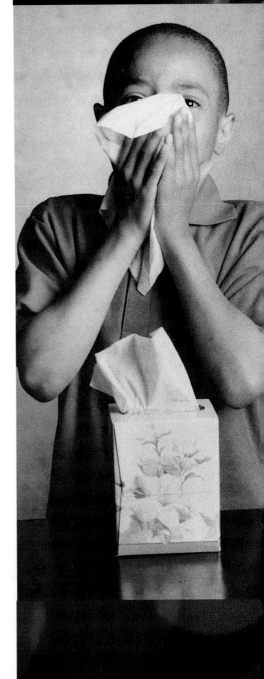

How Do Body Defenses Protect Me?

Body defenses are ways the body works to protect against pathogens. There are two lines of defense. The first line of body defense works against all kinds of pathogens. The second line of body defense works against specific pathogens.

First Line Defenses

Unbroken skin blocks pathogens from entering your body. Help your skin do its job. Wash and cover cuts and scrapes. Bathe or shower daily.

Cilia are tiny hairs that line the air passages. These hairs trap many pathogens and prevent them from entering your lungs. A cough or sneeze forces out the trapped pathogens. Help your cilia do their job. Do not smoke! Smoking paralyzes the cilia. They cannot move and trap germs.

Mucus (MYOO·kuhs) is a moist coating that lines your nose and throat. Mucus helps trap pathogens before they reach your lungs. Help your mucus do its job. Drink plenty of fluids so your nose and throat do not dry out.

Tears coat your eyes each time you blink. Tears wash away dust particles that might contain pathogens. Tears contain a chemical that kills bacteria. Help your tears do their job. Do not rub or irritate your eyes.

Stomach acids can kill pathogens that are swallowed. Help your stomach do its job. Do not drink alcohol. Alcohol irritates the lining of the stomach.

A *white blood cell* is a blood cell that helps destroy pathogens. Help your white blood cells do their job. Get enough rest and sleep. Eat healthful foods, including plenty of vitamin C.

Immunization Schedule

Vaccination and Age Given

Hepatitis B: Birth–2 months, 2–4 months, 6–18 months OR three doses at 11–12 years if not given as an infant

DTP (Diphtheria, **T**etanus, **P**ertussis)**:** 2 months, 4 months, 6 months, 12–18 months, 4–6 years, 11–16 years (DT only)

Hib (Haemophilus **i**nfluenza type **b**)**:** 2 months, 4 months, 6 months, 12–15 months

MMR (Measles, **M**umps, **R**ubella)**:** 12–15 months, 4–6 years, OR 11–12 years

VZ (Varicella **Z**oster-chickenpox)**:** 12–18 months, 11–12 years if not vaccinated or have not had chickenpox

OPV (Oral **P**olio **V**accine)**:** 2 months, 4 months, 6–18 months, 4–6 years

Second Line Defenses

An **antibody** is a substance in the blood that helps fight pathogens. There are different kinds of antibodies in your blood. Each kind works against a certain pathogen.

Suppose you get hepatitis A. Hepatitis A is a mild viral infection of the liver. While you are sick, your body starts producing antibodies to the pathogen that causes hepatitis A. These antibodies stay in your blood even after you become well. They might stay in your blood for the rest of your life. The pathogen that causes hepatitis A might enter your body again. If so, the antibodies to hepatitis A will destroy the pathogen as soon as it enters. You will not become ill with hepatitis A again.

When your body makes antibodies against a certain pathogen, you are immune to that disease. To be **immune** is to be protected from a certain disease. You can also become immune to a disease by getting a vaccine for that disease. A **vaccine** (vak·SEEN) is a medicine that has dead or weak pathogens in it. Pathogens in the vaccine cause your body to produce antibodies for a certain disease. You are then protected from that disease. You might be given a vaccine in a shot or by mouth. There are vaccines for measles, mumps, polio, and flu. Remember to get the necessary vaccines from your doctors or health department.

Pathogen Scrub Off

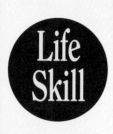

Activity

Life Skill

I will choose habits that prevent the spread of germs.

Materials: Petroleum jelly, sand, soap and water, paper towels

Directions: This activity will help demonstrate the importance of washing your hands to get rid of pathogens.

The Correct Technique for Handwashing

1. **Lather hands with soap and water.**
2. **Rub hands together vigorously for 15 seconds.** Rub the backs of your hands, in between your fingers, and under your nails.
3. **Rinse hands completely under running water.**
4. **Dry your hands with a paper towel.**
5. **Use the paper towel to turn off the faucet.** You might recontaminate your hands if you touch the faucet.

1. **Apply a small amount of petroleum jelly to your hands.**
2. **Rub your hands together and apply the petroleum jelly evenly.** The petroleum jelly represents oils that are present naturally on your skin.
3. **Add a small amount of sand and gently rub your hands together.** The sand represents pathogens on your hands.
4. **Try to wash the sand "pathogens" from your hands using water alone.** Does the water remove the "pathogens"?
5. **Wash your hands with soap and water.** Is it easier to remove the "pathogens"? When you wash your hands, you remove the oil on your skin. The oil contains pathogens, so the pathogens also are removed when you wash.

Handwashing is the single most important way to help prevent the spread of pathogens from person to person. It is important to know the proper handwashing technique to remove pathogens that might be on the skin. Follow The Correct Technique for Handwashing.

Use... Guidelines for Making Responsible Decisions

A friend has invited you to a picnic at her house. You notice a lot of flies crawling on some of the food. The food might be contaminated. Should you eat the food?

Use a separate sheet of paper. Answer "yes" or "no" to each of the following questions. Explain each answer.

1. Is it healthful to eat food that might be contaminated?

2. Is it safe to eat food that might be contaminated?

3. Do you follow rules and laws if you eat food that might be contaminated?

4. Do you show respect for yourself and others if you eat food that might be contaminated?

5. Do you follow your family's guidelines if you eat food that might be contaminated?

6. Do you show good character if you eat food that might be contaminated?

What is the responsible decision to make?

Lesson 28

Review

Vocabulary

Write a separate sentence using each of the vocabulary words listed on page 214.

Health Content

Write answers to the following:

1. What are five kinds of pathogens? **page 215**

2. List six ways pathogens are spread. **pages 216–217**

3. What are ways a person can prevent the spread of pathogens? **page 217**

4. What are ways the body protects a person from pathogens? **pages 218–219**

5. What are ways to help your body defenses do their jobs? **pages 218–219**

Lesson 28 • Stop the Spread of Pathogens **221**

Signs of Sickness

Vocabulary

communicable disease: a disease caused by pathogens that can be spread.

cold: a respiratory infection caused by any of 200 different viruses.

influenza (flu): a viral infection of the respiratory tract.

fever: a higher than normal body temperature.

strep throat: a bacterial infection of the throat.

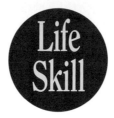

Life Skill

● **I will recognize symptoms and get treatment for communicable diseases.**

Imagine that you touch a wall with wet paint. The paint is now on your hands. It might rub off on everything you touch. You might end up getting paint on many different surfaces. Like the paint, communicable diseases can be spread to many other objects and people.

A **communicable disease** is a disease caused by pathogens that can be spread. You can choose behaviors to reduce your risk of becoming infected with pathogens. You can choose behaviors to reduce the risk of spreading pathogens.

The Lesson Objectives

● Define communicable disease.

● List the three stages of disease.

● Discuss the symptoms of and treatments for communicable diseases.

● Tell ways to reduce the risk of getting a cold, the flu, or a sore throat.

What Are the Stages of Disease?

Suppose a pathogen enters your body. Your body defenses might destroy the pathogen. The pathogen might not multiply. You might never have symptoms of illness. You might not have to stay home from school and recover. This is what happens most of the time. But what happens when you do get sick? What are the stages of disease?

The *incubation period* is the time between when a pathogen enters the body until symptoms of disease appear. During this period, the pathogen multiplies. This period can last from a few hours or days to a few weeks or longer. Your body will try to destroy the pathogens during this time. This is why you always need to be in the best health you can be.

The *acute period* is the time during which symptoms of disease are the greatest. Suppose you have a cold. The acute period begins with the first sneeze. You are very contagious at this time. The length of the acute period varies. It depends on how well your body fights off the disease. This is why you need to drink plenty of water and get rest and sleep. You must give your body every chance to fight the disease.

The *recovery period* is the time during which visible symptoms of disease go away but you are not back to full speed. You might still be able to spread pathogens during this period. A carrier of disease is a person who does not have symptoms but can still spread pathogens. Your general health affects how long the recovery period lasts. You can relapse or go back to the acute period if you try to do too much too soon.

Give Yourself a Chance for Full Recovery

Suppose you have had a bad cold or flu. You have been absent from school for several days. When you return to school, pamper yourself for a few days. Rest after school. Do not push yourself. Do not return to hard workouts too soon. Get plenty of sleep. This helps prevent a relapse. A relapse is when you get the symptoms for the same disease again. There is another reason to pamper yourself. Your body is not back to full speed. There will be pathogens at your school. During the recovery period, you might get other pathogens in your body. If you do not take care of yourself, you can get sick again.

How Can I Reduce My Risk of Getting a Cold ?

A **cold** is a respiratory infection caused by any of 200 different viruses. Symptoms might include sneezing, a runny, stuffy nose, watery eyes, headache, and perhaps a cough. Colds usually stay in the head, throat, or chest. The cold is the most common communicable disease. Most people your age have at least two colds each year. For this reason, the cold is often referred to as the "common cold."

There is no cure for a cold. Be sure to rest and drink plenty of fluids. There are over-the-counter (OTC) drugs that can help relieve symptoms.

There are ways to reduce your risk of getting a cold.

- Wash your hands with soap and water often.
- Avoid close contact with people who have colds and any objects they touch.
- Keep your fingers and other objects out of your eyes, nose, and mouth.
- Do not get too close to a person who is coughing or sneezing. Colds are spread by breathing in droplets from an infected person.

Do not spread the cold virus to others. Do not touch others or let people use objects that might contain your pathogens. Cover your coughs and sneezes. Your parents or guardian might decide to keep you home from school if you have a cold.

Your parents or guardian caution you to take it easy when you have a cold. Your body is trying to recover from being infected with the cold virus. During recovery, it is easier for other pathogens to multiply in your body. For example, it is easier for you to get flu.

Trap a Cough or Sneeze with a Tissue

Suppose you have a bad cold and cough and sneeze. Try to use a tissue to trap your cough and sneeze. Put the used tissue in a garbage bag. Do not keep a used tissue. Remember, it has been used to trap your cough and sneeze. There will be pathogens on it. After you cough or sneeze, wash your hands with soap and water.

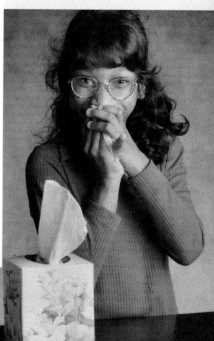

How Can I Reduce My Risk of Getting the Flu?

Influenza (in·floo·EN·zuh) or **flu** is a viral infection of the respiratory tract. Symptoms of flu include body aches, chills, headache, cough, chest discomfort, tiredness, and fever. **Fever** is a higher than normal body temperature. Symptoms of flu are more severe than those of the common cold.

There is no cure for the flu. Get plenty of rest and drink plenty of fluids. Over-the-counter drugs can help relieve symptoms, but it is important to ask your doctor which products to use. Taking aspirin might cause Reye's syndrome. Reye's syndrome is a disorder that causes brain and liver damage.

There are ways to reduce your risk of getting the flu.

- Wash your hands with soap and water often.
- Avoid close contact with people who have the flu and any objects they touch.
- Keep your fingers and other objects out of your eyes, nose, and mouth.
- Do not get near a person who is coughing or sneezing. The flu is spread by breathing droplets from an infected person.
- Get the flu vaccine if a doctor recommends it. A new vaccine must be given each year because the virus changes each year.

Do not spread the flu virus to others. Do not get close to others. Do not touch others or let people use objects that might contain your pathogens. Cover your coughs and sneezes. Your parents or guardian might decide to keep you home from school if you have the flu.

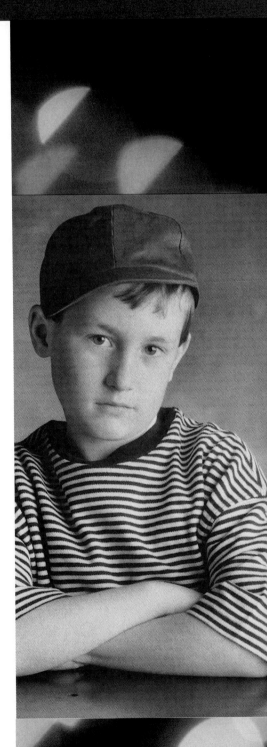

How Can I Reduce My Risk of Getting a Sore Throat?

A *sore throat* is a sore or scratchy throat. It can be caused by a bacterial infection, a viral infection, or irritation from post-nasal drip from allergies or a cold. **Strep throat** is a bacterial infection of the throat. Symptoms might include extreme soreness of the throat, difficulty in swallowing, fever, and muscle aches. Your doctor might prescribe antibiotics. It is important to finish all antibiotics even if you begin to feel better. Untreated strep throat can cause permanent heart damage.

If you do not have strep throat but your throat is sore, your sore throat is probably caused by a virus. Fever and muscle aches might also be present. Antibiotics are not prescribed for a sore throat caused by a virus. Treatment includes drinking plenty of fluids and getting plenty of rest. Ask your doctor which over-the-counter drugs might be taken.

There are ways to reduce your risk of getting a sore throat.

- Wash your hands with soap and water often.
- Avoid close contact with people who have strep throat and any objects they touch.

Note: People who have strep throat usually are not contagious after one or two days of taking antibiotics.

- Keep your fingers and other objects out of your eyes, nose, and mouth.
- Do not get near a person who is coughing or sneezing. Sore throats are spread by breathing in droplets from an infected person.

Do not touch others or let people use objects that might contain your pathogens. Cover your coughs and sneezes. Your parents or guardian might decide to keep you home from school if you have a sore throat.

Lyme Disease

Lyme disease is a bacterial infection spread by ticks. A tick is an insect that attaches to humans and animals. Ticks that spread Lyme disease attach to field mice and deer. Then the ticks attach to the human body and bite to get blood. Bacteria enter the body. A rash results that grows to be about seven inches across. The center of the rash is light red. The outer ridges are darker red and raised. Other symptoms include fever, headache, and weakness. See a doctor right away if these symptoms appear. Antibiotics are needed. Reduce the risk of getting Lyme disease. Keep ticks off your body. Wear long clothing when you are in the woods or fields. Wear a lotion that keeps ticks off the body. Check your body for ticks after being in woods and fields.

Use... Guidelines for Making Responsible Decisions™

A friend has invited you to join him on a camping trip. In your gear you have included long pants, shirts with long sleeves, and socks to cover and protect your body from ticks when in the woods or fields. You also have taken a special lotion that helps keep ticks off your body. Your friend says this isn't necessary and not to worry. He says he isn't going to do anything to protect himself. Should he protect himself?

Use a separate sheet of paper. Answer "yes" or "no" to each of the following questions. Explain each answer.

1. Is it healthful for your friend not to protect himself?
2. Is it safe for your friend not to protect himself?
3. Does your friend follow rules and laws if he does not protect himself?
4. Does your friend show respect for himself and others if he does not protect himself?
5. Does your friend follow his family's guidelines if he does not protect himself?
6. Does your friend show good character if he does not protect himself?

What is the responsible decision to make?

Lesson 29

Review

Vocabulary

Write a separate sentence using each of the vocabulary words listed on page 222.

Health Content

Write answers to the following:

1. What are the three stages of disease? **page 223**
2. List the symptoms and treatment for a cold. **page 224**
3. List the symptoms and treatment for the flu. **page 225**
4. List the symptoms and treatment for strep throat. **page 226**
5. What are ways to reduce your risk of getting a cold, the flu, or a sore throat? **pages 224–226**

Don't Risk Heart Disease and Cancer

Vocabulary

heart disease: a disease of the heart and blood vessels.

angina pectoris: chest pain caused by a lack of oxygen in the heart.

heart attack: a sudden lack of oxygen to the heart.

premature heart disease: heart disease that occurs before old age.

cancer: a disease in which cells multiply in ways that are not normal.

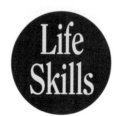

Life Skills

- I will choose habits that prevent heart disease.
- I will choose habits that prevent cancer.

Your habits now affect your future health. If you have healthful habits now you can reduce the risk of getting some diseases later. You can protect yourself against heart disease and cancer.

The Lesson Objectives

- Discuss different kinds of heart disease.
- Discuss habits that protect against premature heart disease.
- List the warning signs for cancer.
- Discuss habits that protect against cancer.

What Are Different Kinds of Heart Disease?

Heart disease is a disease of the heart and blood vessels. Heart disease is one of the leading causes of death. There are many kinds of heart disease.

Congenital (kuhn·JEN·uh·tuhl) *heart disease* is defects in the heart that are present at birth. The anatomy of the heart might not be as it should. For example, the walls might not be formed the right way. The valves of the heart or the blood vessels might not be formed the right way. These defects can change the way blood flows. For example, blood might not flow to the lungs to get oxygen. Surgery is used to correct the defects. A baby might have surgery shortly after birth.

Rheumatic (roo·MAT·ik) *heart disease* is damage to the heart valves that occurs if strep throat is not treated. Suppose you have a very bad sore throat. You need to have a throat culture to learn if you have strep throat. Your doctor can prescribe antibiotics or other drugs. These drugs kill the bacteria which cause strep throat.

Suppose you do not get treatment for strep throat. You might get rheumatic fever. The symptoms are fever, weakness, and swelling around body joints. This leads to damage to heart valves. Then you have rheumatic heart disease.

What Is a Heart Murmur?

A doctor listens to the heart with a stethoscope. The sounds the doctor hears are caused by the opening and closing of the heart valves. A heart murmur is abnormal sound from the opening and closing of valves. Some heart murmurs are serious, while others are not. For example, a damaged valve might cause heart murmur. Surgery might be needed. Harmless heart murmurs are common in children. They are caused by the rapid flow of blood through small structures in the heart.

Angina pectoris (an·JY·nuh PEK·tuhr·uhs) is chest pain caused by a lack of oxygen in the heart. This might result from a buildup of fatty materials in the blood vessels. The blood vessels that supply the heart become narrow. Enough blood cannot travel to the heart. Angina occurs most often during times of stress or exercise. Sometimes the pain will spread from the heart to the arm. The pain goes away when the person stops exercising or the stress is gone.

A doctor might give the person medicine that can cause the blood vessels in the heart to open wider. This allows more blood to enter the heart.

A **heart attack** is a sudden lack of oxygen to the heart. A heart attack usually happens because an artery is blocked or gets narrow. Arteries become blocked when fatty materials collect on the artery walls. Blood flow is reduced. Blood carries oxygen to the heart. If a large area of the heart muscle cannot get oxygen, serious damage can occur.

Usually the first sign of a heart attack is pain. The pain is strongest in the center of the chest. The pain is often felt in the shoulder, neck, jaw, and arms. The person might have trouble breathing. The person might have cold, pale skin. This happens because the heart is not pumping enough blood to the body parts. The person might vomit. The pain of a heart attack is not relieved by rest. If you notice any of these symptoms in a person, get help immediately. The sooner a person gets help, the better the chance for recovery.

High Blood Pressure

High blood pressure increases the chance of a heart attack. High blood pressure is the force of blood against artery walls. If the force is too great, artery walls are damaged. It is easier for fatty materials to build up inside artery walls. Children can have high blood pressure. Your doctor will measure your blood pressure when you have a checkup. Follow your doctor's advice if you have high blood pressure.

What Habits Protect Me from Premature Heart Disease?

People who have reached old age might develop heart disease. Their heart and blood vessels have worked for years. At some time in life, they will not function as well. **Premature heart disease** is heart disease that occurs before old age. Your habits now can keep you from having premature heart disease.

Follow these habits to protect against premature heart disease.

- **Get plenty of physical activity.** Physical activity helps keep your heart strong. Physical activity helps you maintain a healthful weight. It lowers your body fat. It helps clear fat from the blood, and reduces the effects of stress. Activities such as walking, running, riding a bike, aerobics, and swimming can help keep the heart healthy.

- **Handle stress in a healthful manner**. Talk with someone if you have a problem. Being stressed causes the heart to work harder than it should. You might become tired, but not be able to rest well. Your heart does not get the rest it needs. Stress management skills help you cope with body changes stress can cause.

- **Do not smoke!** Cigarette smoking is the greatest risk factor for developing premature heart disease. The risk is 70 percent higher for a smoker than a nonsmoker. By not smoking, you allow your heart to get the oxygen it needs. The heart is not overworked due to lack of oxygen.

- **Cut back on fat.** Diets high in fats increase the risk of premature heart disease. Eat foods such as salads, fruits, vegetables, and fish. Eating these kinds of foods will help prevent a buildup of fats in your blood vessels.

- **Stay at a healthful weight.** Lose weight if you are overweight. The heart must work harder to pump blood to the various parts of the body if a person is overweight.

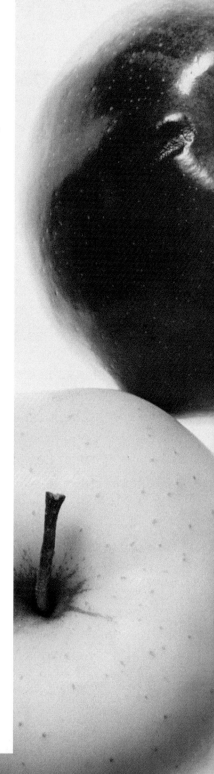

What Habits Protect Me from Cancer?

Cancer is a disease in which cells multiply in ways that are not normal. Many kinds of cancer can be prevented. Some are caused by harmful habits. The cause of other kinds is unknown. The earlier cancer is found, the easier it might be to treat. Choose habits that reduce your risk of cancer.

Do not use tobacco products. Tobacco is the number one cause of cancers of the lungs, mouth, throat, and digestive system. Smoking is the most important risk factor you can control. There would be fewer cases of lung cancer if people did not smoke. Smoking as a teen can increase the risk of cancer later in life. For example, breast cancer is more common in females who smoked as teens. Other tobacco products also increase cancer risk. Smokeless tobacco increases the risk of cancers of the mouth, gums, and throat. These cancers can develop within a few years of use.

Use a sunscreen with an SPF of 15 or more. Exposure to ultraviolet (UV) radiation is the main cause of skin cancer. Know how to protect yourself. Wear a sunscreen with a sun protection factor (SPF) of 15 or more. The sun's harmful rays are most powerful between 10:00 a.m. and 4:00 p.m. Avoid being in the sun during these hours. If you are in the sun, cover exposed body parts. Know that certain medications, such as some antibiotics, can increase the chance of sunburn. It is also important to wear sunglasses that protect against UV radiation. Do not use tanning booths or sun lamps. Check your skin regularly for signs of skin cancer. Signs of skin cancer are certain changes of the skin, moles, or a sore that does not heal. If you notice any growths on your skin that do not appear normal, see your doctor.

Limit the amount of fat you eat. A diet high in fat has been linked to breast, colon, and prostate cancers. Check the nutrition label on food products. Cut back on foods you eat that are high in fat.

Eat plenty of fruits and vegetables. Eat five or more servings of fruits and vegetables a day. They provide fiber. Fiber helps reduce your risk of colon cancer. Fruits and vegetables also contain antioxidants, such as vitamins A, C, and E. Antioxidants are substances that help prevent cancer. Fruits and vegetables are also low in calories and help you maintain a desirable weight.

Do not breathe fumes from products with harmful chemicals, such as some household products. Exposure to household chemicals increases your risk of certain cancers. Wear rubber gloves and a mask when using cleaning products or insect sprays. Use glues, paints, and thinners in areas that are well-ventilated.

See a doctor if you have a warning sign of cancer. It is important to know the warning signs of cancer. Cancers are easier to treat if discovered early. Having one of these signs does not always mean you have cancer. Your doctor can determine the reason for your symptoms. Remember the word CAUTION.

Change in bowel or bladder habits

A sore that does not heal

Unusual bleeding or discharge

Thickening or lump in the breast or elsewhere

Indigestion or difficulty in swallowing

Obvious change in a wart or mole

Nagging cough or hoarseness

Healthy Heart Hop

Activity

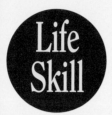

Life Skill

I will choose habits that protect against heart disease.

Materials: Two large blank index cards, red and blue markers; access to the playground or gym, chalk

Directions: Review risk behaviors and healthful behaviors for heart disease.

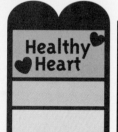

Healthy Heart

Start

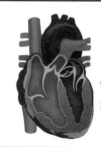

I ride my bicycle after school.

Heart Healthful Behavior Card

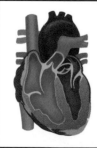

I am a couch potato.

Heart Risk Behavior Card

1. **Make a Heart Healthful Behavior card.** Look at the illustration. Use an index card. Use the red and blue markers to draw a heart like the one that is shown. Then write a healthful behavior for your heart. On the other side of the card, write a number from one to five.

2. **Make a Heart Risk Behavior card.** Follow the instructions for step one but write a risk behavior on an index card.

3. **Use chalk to draw a path with spaces on it (see the illustration).** There should be at least 35 spaces.

4. **Shuffle the cards and place them in a pile.**

5. **Form a line at the start and begin the Heart Healthy Hop.** One classmate begins. The teacher will read the number and the behavior on the first card in the pile. For example, the teacher will say, "Three spaces. I will ride my bicycle after school." This is a heart healthful behavior card. The classmate who begins will hop forward three spaces. If the first card is a heart risk behavior card, the classmate does not begin. If a classmate has hopped forward on the path and draws a heart risk behavior card, the classmate must hop backwards. The game ends when a student reaches the healthy heart.

A friend of yours is going to a tanning booth to keep her tan year round. She suggests that you also would look healthier with a tan. Should you start using a tanning booth?

Use a separate sheet of paper. Answer "yes" or "no" to each of the following questions. Explain each answer.

1. Is it healthful for you to use a tanning booth?
2. Is it safe for you to use a tanning booth?
3. Do you follow rules and laws if you use a tanning booth?
4. Do you show respect for yourself and others if you use a tanning booth?
5. Do you follow your family's guidelines if you use a tanning booth?
6. Do you show good character if you use a tanning booth?

What is the responsible decision to make?

Lesson 30

Review

Vocabulary

Write a separate sentence using each of the vocabulary words listed on page 228.

Health Content

Write answers to the following:

1. How is congenital heart disease treated?
   page 229
2. What are two kinds of heart disease that are caused by habits? What are signs of a heart attack? **page 230**
3. What are habits to protect against premature heart disease? **page 231**
4. What are five habits to protect against cancer?
   pages 232–233
5. What are the seven warning signs of cancer?
   page 233

Caring for Chronic Health Conditions

Vocabulary

chronic health condition: a condition that lasts a long time or keeps coming back.

allergy: the reaction of the body to certain substances.

asthma: a chronic disease in which the small airways get narrow.

epilepsy: a chronic disease in which nerve messages in the brain are disturbed for brief periods of time.

diabetes: a disease in which the body does not make or cannot use insulin.

arthritis: the painful swelling of joints in the body.

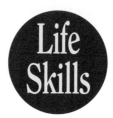
Life Skills

- I will tell ways to care for allergies and asthma.
- I will tell ways to care for chronic (lasting) health conditions.

Many young people have a chronic health condition. A **chronic health conditon** is a condition that lasts a long time or keeps coming back. Some of these diseases might be present at birth. Others might develop during a person's life. There are many ways to treat these diseases. People with chronic diseases live healthful lives.

The Lesson Objectives

- Describe what happens when a person has allergies.
- Tell ways a person can manage asthma.
- Explain how to help a person who is having a seizure.
- Discuss causes and treatment for diabetes.
- Discuss ways to care for chronic health conditions.

What Is an Allergy?

An **allergy** (Al·uhr·jee) is the reaction of the body to certain substances. An *allergen* is a substance that causes an allergic reaction.

Some allergens are dog and cat dander, grass, molds, pollen, and dust. Common food allergens are milk, eggs, nuts, wheat, corn, tomatoes, and shellfish.

The body mistakes an allergen for a harmful invader. Chemical substances are released from cells in the body. These chemical substances cause symptoms to appear.

Symptoms for allergies vary among people. They might include sneezing, runny nose, and watery, itchy eyes. A person might have a stuffed-up feeling in the nose, ears, and chest. There might be headaches, hives, and a feeling of itchiness. Some people have severe reactions to allergens. These symptoms might include dizziness, nausea, skin rash, drop in blood pressure, and difficulty in breathing. In these cases, immediate medical attention is needed. People with very bad allergies might carry special medications with them.

An *allergist* is a doctor who treats people with allergies. The allergist might test a person for different allergens. The allergens are placed in the body through small scratches in the skin. The allergist checks for the reactions to the different allergens. Treatments might be prescribed. The treatments reduce a person's reaction to an allergen. Sometimes treatments cause the reaction to disappear.

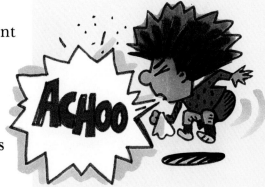

What Is Asthma?

Asthma (AZ·muh) is a chronic disease in which the small airways get narrow. Asthma triggers are substances or conditions that can cause asthma attacks. Common asthma triggers include animal dander, dust and mold, pollen, colognes, cold air, cigarette smoke, stress, vigorous exercise, tiredness, household cleaning products, aspirin, and other over-the-counter (OTC) drugs.

An asthma attack is an episode of coughing, wheezing, and shortness of breath. Breathing might be so difficult that first aid is needed. Other signs and symptoms of an asthma attack might include itchy or sore throat, rapid breathing, and tightness in the chest.

Asthma attacks often happen at night when a person is lying down resting or sleeping. When in this position, mucus does not drain as well from the air passages. Mucus can build up in the air passages. Most attacks are mild. In a severe attack, a person will struggle to breathe. He or she might have to go to the hospital.

Asthma cannot be cured, but it can be controlled. Young people with asthma must work with a doctor to get treatment. Avoid asthma triggers. Follow all advice from a doctor and take medications that might be prescribed for you. Check with your doctor before taking over-the-counter (OTC) medicine. Some people with asthma use an inhaler to get medicine into air passages and lungs. Know when and how to get medical help for severe asthma attacks.

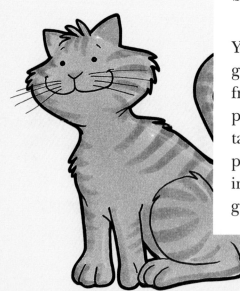

What Are Epilepsy and Diabetes?

Epilepsy (EP·uh·LEP·see) is a chronic disease in which nerve messages in the brain are disturbed for brief periods of time. Epilepsy might be caused by an injury to the head. It might also be caused by lack of oxygen to the brain. In many cases, the causes are unknown. This disease results in a temporary loss of control of thinking and muscular movement. The person might have a seizure. A *seizure* (SEE·zhuhr) is the period of time during which loss of control occurs.

Most seizures are not serious. During a seizure, a person should be watched to be sure he or she is not injured. Often the seizure will last less than one minute. Sometimes the person might twitch and shake. Try to keep the person free from injury by removing nearby objects. Do not try to stop the person from moving during the seizure. Let the person rest after the seizure.

People with epilepsy can be treated with medicine. The medicine will help reduce the number of seizures a person will have.

Diabetes (DY·uh·BEE·teez) is a disease in which the body does not make or cannot use insulin. The *pancreas* (PAN·kree·us) is a gland that produces insulin. *Insulin* is a hormone that helps body cells use sugar from foods. Body cells use sugar to release energy. Some people with diabetes produce little or no insulin. Other people with diabetes produce insulin, but it does not work well. In either case, their body cells cannot use sugar.

When diabetes occurs in young children, little or no insulin is produced in the body. A person who has this type of diabetes must have shots of insulin daily. They must also follow a special diet of foods low in sugar.

The other form of diabetes occurs in adulthood. In this kind, some insulin is produced but might not work well. This type of diabetes can usually be controlled through diet and exercise or medicine.

What Are Other Chronic Diseases?

There are many other chronic health conditions. *Cerebral palsy* (suh·REE·bruhl PAHL·zee) is a chronic disease that interferes with muscle coordination. A person with cerebral palsy might have a hard time standing or walking. The person might have difficulty speaking, hearing, and seeing. These symptoms remain through life. Mental skills are usually not affected. Treatment includes physical therapy and speech therapy. Surgery might help in some cases.

Arthritis (ar·THRY·tis) is the painful swelling of joints in the body. One kind of arthritis is caused by wear and tear on joints. Sports injuries, being overweight, and heredity can be factors. Another kind of arthritis involves joint deformity. Treatment consists of pain relievers and certain exercises to help improve movement of the joint area. Sometimes surgery is performed to replace joints.

Cystic fibrosis (sis·tik fy·BROH·sis) is an inherited disease in which thick mucus clogs the lungs. Body organs can be damaged by these large amounts of mucus. Signs and symptoms of cystic fibrosis include coughing, wheezing, difficulty breathing, vomiting, and constipation. Cystic fibrosis is caused by an abnormal gene. Treatment might include medications, physical therapy, changes in diet, vitamins, and oxygen to help with breathing.

Muscular dystrophy (DIS·truh·fee) is a disease in which muscles lose the ability to work. Muscular dystrophy is rare. The most common type affects males. There is no cure. Treatment might include physical therapy and physical activity to keep muscles in good condition. Weight management is also important to keep joints healthy.

It is important to be aware of various chronic health conditions. It is important to understand and appreciate the special needs of people that have these conditions. They do not let their diseases stop them from doing what they want to do.

Use... Guidelines for Making Responsible Decisions™

A group of friends has invited you to go on a hiking trip this weekend. **?** At this time of year, the pollen count is very high. You have asthma and you know that the pollen might bring on an asthma attack. But you don't pack your inhaler because you don't want to look like a geek.

Use a separate sheet of paper. Answer "yes" or "no" to each of the following questions. Explain each answer.

1. Is it healthful not to pack your inhaler?
2. Is it safe not to pack your inhaler?
3. Do you follow rules and laws if you do not pack your inhaler?
4. Do you show respect for yourself and others if you do not pack your inhaler?
5. Do you follow your family's guidelines if you do not pack your inhaler?
6. Do you show good character if you do not pack your inhaler?

What is the responsible decision to make?

Lesson 31

Review

Vocabulary

Write a separate sentence using each of the vocabulary words listed on page 236.

Health Content

Write answers to the following:

1. How does the body react to allergens? **page 237**
2. What are five common asthma triggers? **page 238**
3. What are three actions to take when a person has a seizure? **page 239**
4. List the causes and treatments for diabetes. **page 239**
5. What is the cause and treatment for cerebral palsy? **page 240**

HIV and AIDS: The Facts

Vocabulary

helper T cell: a white blood cell that helps make antibodies.

HIV: the virus that destroys helper T cells and causes AIDS.

AIDS: a breakdown in the body's ability to fight infection.

opportunistic disease: a disease that would not occur if the body defenses were working.

universal precautions: steps taken to keep from having contact with pathogens in body fluids.

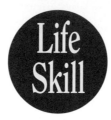

Life Skill

● **I will learn facts about HIV and AIDS.**

HIV is a virus. If a person gets HIV he or she will have it forever. The person will get AIDS. This lesson gives the facts about HIV and AIDS. You will learn how HIV gets into the body. You will learn ways to keep HIV out of the body. Then you can choose responsible behaviors.

The Lesson Objectives

● Discuss how HIV infection leads to AIDS.

● Tell ways HIV is spread.

● Tell ways HIV is not spread.

● List ways to prevent HIV infection.

How Does HIV Infection Lead to AIDS?

Every day pathogens enter your body. Most of the time you stay well. This is because your body is able to fight pathogens. Certain cells in your body help fight pathogens. A **helper T cell** is a white blood cell that helps make antibodies. An *antibody* is a substance in the blood that helps fight pathogens. You have large numbers of helper T cells in your body.

Suppose pathogens enter your body. Helper T cells go to work. They tell your body to make antibodies to fight the pathogens. Then the pathogens cannot make you sick. Antibodies can be made to fight many different kinds of pathogens.

But something different happens when HIV enters the body. **HIV** is a virus that destroys helper T cells and causes AIDS. When HIV enters the body, HIV finds the helper T cells. It gets inside the helper T cells and destroys them. Then there are fewer helper T cells to tell the body to make antibodies.

A person who is infected with HIV gets weaker as the number of helper T cells gets lower. After a period of time, a person will have AIDS. **AIDS** is a breakdown in the body's ability to fight infection. A person has AIDS when:

- the number of helper T cells in the blood is low;
- a blood test shows antibodies for HIV;
- opportunistic diseases are present.

An **opportunistic** (AHP·uhr·too·NIST·ik) **disease** is a disease that would not occur if body defenses were working normally. These diseases have the "opportunity" to occur because the body is so weak. One of these is a special kind of pneumonia. Another is a type of skin cancer that causes purple blotches on the skin.

A Quick Review

- HIV enters the body.
- HIV clings to helper T cells and destroys some of them. There are fewer helper T cells to tell the body to make antibodies.
- HIV multiplies. The additional HIV destroys even more helper T cells. There are even fewer helper T cells to tell the body to make antibodies.
- A person has AIDS when: the number of helper T cells is very low; a blood test shows antibodies for HIV; opportunistic diseases are present.

What Are Ways HIV Is Spread?

Suppose a person is infected with HIV. A person who is infected with HIV has HIV in his or her body fluids. The person might not even know that he or she is infected. If you have contact with this person's body fluids, you can become infected with HIV.

A *risk behavior* is an action that can be harmful to you and others. There are risk behaviors for HIV. These risk behaviors increase the chance that you will have contact with body fluids that have HIV.

- Not sticking to your decision to practice abstinence
- Sharing a needle to inject drugs with a person who has HIV
- Sharing a needle to pierce ears or other body parts with a person who has HIV
- Sharing a needle for tattooing with a person who has HIV
- Pricking your finger and rubbing blood together to become a blood brother or sister with a person who has HIV
- Touching the blood from a nosebleed or cut of a person who has HIV

What Are Ways HIV Is Not Spread?

HIV is not spread by casual contact. *Casual contact* is daily contact without touching body fluids. Some kinds of casual contact are shaking hands, using the same pencil, holding hands, and hugging. To date, HIV has not been spread by breathing moist droplets from someone's sneeze or cough. You cannot get HIV by sitting next to a classmate who is infected.

Blood Transfusions

Suppose a person needs the blood of another person. The person might have an operation and need blood. The person might have a health condition and need blood. The person needing blood gets a blood transfusion. In the past, some people who had blood transfusions were given blood that had HIV in it. They did not know it when they got the blood transfusion. Today, there are tests to check out blood to keep it from being used if it has HIV in it.

What Are Ways to Prevent HIV Infection?

There is no cure for AIDS right now. There are medicines that keep people who have AIDS alive as long as possible. Scientists are working to find new drugs. They are working on vaccines to keep people from getting AIDS. They want to find a cure.

You can choose behaviors to keep from getting infected with HIV. You can stay away from risk behaviors. Here are actions you can take.

- Practice abstinence.
- Do not use a needle and inject drugs.
- Do not share a needle and pierce your ears or other body parts. Get permission from your parents or guardian if you want to have ears pierced. If they say NO, do what they say. If they say YES, they can be certain it is done right. Sterile equipment will be used. Get permission from your parents or guardian for body piercing. If they say NO, do what they say.
- Do not share a needle for a tattoo. Do not get a tattoo without the permission of your parents or guardian. Know that many people regret having gotten a tattoo.
- Do not prick your finger and rub blood to become a blood brother or sister.
- Do not touch the blood of a person who has a nosebleed, cut, or other injury.

Suppose you are on the playground. A classmate is struck in the face by a rubber ball. Your classmate has a nosebleed. Get your teacher or the teacher who is watching the playground to help. A teacher will have a kit with throw-away latex gloves in it. A teacher will wear the throw-away latex gloves while he or she helps your classmate.

Drinking Alcohol Can Cause You to Make Wrong Decisions

Do not drink alcohol. It is against the law for you to drink. Alcohol slows down the brain cells. You do not think clearly. You might not think about facts. You might not consider actions to stay healthy. Drinking alcohol might cause you to choose risk behaviors. Certain risk behaviors can result in getting HIV.

Universal Caution Protection

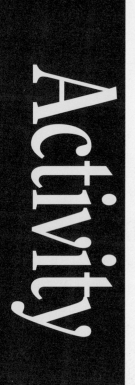

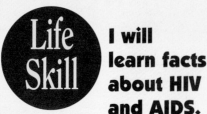

I will learn facts about HIV and AIDS.

Materials: Throw-away latex gloves, cup of water, red and yellow food coloring, bowl, paper towels

Directions: Read the box to learn about universal precautions. Complete this activity to learn why a teacher or coach wears throw-away latex gloves if you or a classmate is injured.

Universal Precautions

Universal precautions are steps taken to keep from having contact with pathogens in body fluids. Health care workers such as your doctor and dentist take these steps. Your teachers and coaches take these steps. You must take these steps if you help someone who is bleeding.

- Wear throw-away latex gloves.
- Wear the gloves only one time.
- Wash your hands with soap and water when you take the gloves off.
- Do not eat or drink anything while you help someone who is bleeding.
- Do not touch your mouth, eyes, or nose while you help the person.

1. **Put several drops of red food coloring in the cup of water to make "blood."**

2. **Pretend the yellow food coloring is blood from someone who has HIV.** With your classmates, list the ways that HIV is spread.

3. **Add a drop of yellow food coloring to the cup of red water to make blood with HIV in it.** Pretend this is the blood of a person who is infected with HIV.

4. **Ask a classmate to volunteer.** Have the classmate place a hand over the bowl. Pretend the classmate has at least one cut on the hand. Pour some of the blood with HIV in it on his or her hand. It will run off into the bowl. How could the HIV get into your classmate's body?

5. **Ask another classmate to volunteer and wear the throw-away latex gloves.** Pretend the classmate has at least one cut on the hand. Pour some of the blood with HIV in it on his or her hand. It will run off into the bowl. How did this classmate keep HIV out of his or her body?

Use... Guidelines for Making Responsible Decisions™

You meet three new friends at camp. They want to seal the friendship. They want to prick their finger and have it bleed. Then you will rub your fingers together. They say this is how to become a blood brother or sister.

Use a separate sheet of paper. Answer "yes" or "no" to each of the following questions. Explain each answer.

1. Is it healthful to touch the blood of your new friends?

2. Is it safe to touch the blood of your new friends?

3. Do you follow rules and laws if you touch the blood of your new friends?

4. Do you show respect for yourself and others if you touch the blood of your new friends?

5. Do you follow your family's guidelines if you touch the blood of your new friends?

6. Do you show good character if you touch the blood of your new friends?

What is the responsible decision to make?

Lesson 32

Review

Vocabulary

Write a separate sentence using each of the vocabulary words listed on page 242.

Health Content

Write answers to the following:

1. How does HIV infection lead to AIDS? **page 243**

2. What are ways HIV is spread? **page 244**

3. What are ways HIV is not spread? **page 244**

4. What are ways to prevent HIV infection? **page 245**

5. What are universal precautions to take if you help someone who is bleeding? **page 246**

Unit 7 Review

Health Content

Review your answers for each Lesson Review in this unit. Write answers to the following questions.

1. What actions can you take to prevent the spread of pathogens? **Lesson 28 page 217**

2. What are first line defenses that protect you from pathogens? **Lesson 28 page 218**

3. How is the flu treated? **Lesson 29 page 225**

4. What are symptoms of strep throat? **Lesson 29 page 226**

5. What can happen to your heart if you do not get treated for strep throat? **Lesson 30 page 229**

6. How does eating fruits and vegetables help protect against cancer? **Lesson 30 page 233**

7. What are symptoms of an allergy? **Lesson 31 page 237**

8. How is cerebral palsy treated? **Lesson 31 page 240**

9. What actions can you take to keep from getting infected with HIV? **Lesson 32 page 245**

10. How should you protect yourself if you help someone who is bleeding? **Lesson 32 page 246**

Guidelines for Making Responsible Decisions™

A classmate has cerebral palsy. The person has a hard time walking. Sometimes other classmates make fun of this person. Use a separate sheet of paper. Answer "yes" or "no" to each of the following questions. Explain each answer.

1. Is it healthful to make fun of a person who has a chronic health condition?

2. Is it safe to make fun of a person who has a chronic health condition?

3. Do you follow rules and laws if you make fun of a person who has a chronic health condition?

4. Do you show respect for yourself and others if you make fun of a person who has a chronic health condition?

5. Do you follow your family's guidelines if you make fun of a person who has a chronic health condition?

6. Do you show good character if you make fun of a person who has a chronic health condition?

What is the responsible decision to make?

Family Involvement

Have your family help you write humorous reminders to family members to wash their hands. Tape the cards in the kitchen and bathroom.

Vocabulary

Number a sheet of paper from 1–10. Read each definition. Next to each number on your sheet of paper, write the vocabulary word that matches the definition.

angina pectoris	fever
antibody	influenza
premature heart disease	arthritis
universal precautions	epilepsy
helper T cell	virus

1. A viral infection of the respiratory tract. **Lesson 29**
2. A white blood cell that helps make antibodies. **Lesson 32**
3. Chest pain caused by a lack of oxygen in the heart. **Lesson 30**
4. Heart disease that occurs before old age. **Lesson 30**
5. A chronic disease in which nerve messages in the brain are disturbed for brief periods of time. **Lesson 31**
6. Steps taken to keep from having contact with pathogens in body fluids. **Lesson 32**
7. A pathogen that makes copies of itself. **Lesson 28**
8. A higher than normal body temperature. **Lesson 29**
9. A substance in the blood that helps fight pathogens. **Lesson 28**
10. The painful swelling of joints in the body. **Lesson 31**

SPEEDWAY PUBLIC LIBRARY
SPEEDWAY, INDIANA

Health Literacy

Effective Communication

 Use the word "communicable." Make up tips for preventing colds that begin with each letter.

Self-Directed Learning

 Call or write your local chapter of the American Heart Association. Ask them to mail you information on heart by-pass surgery.

Critical Thinking

 Why might a person who abuses drugs be more likely to get infected with HIV?

Responsible Citizenship

 Talk with a student who has a chronic disease. Ask the student how other students can show respect and understanding. Share the answers with your class.

Multicultural Health

Compare the number of deaths from lung cancer in your country to that of another country. What might cause any difference?

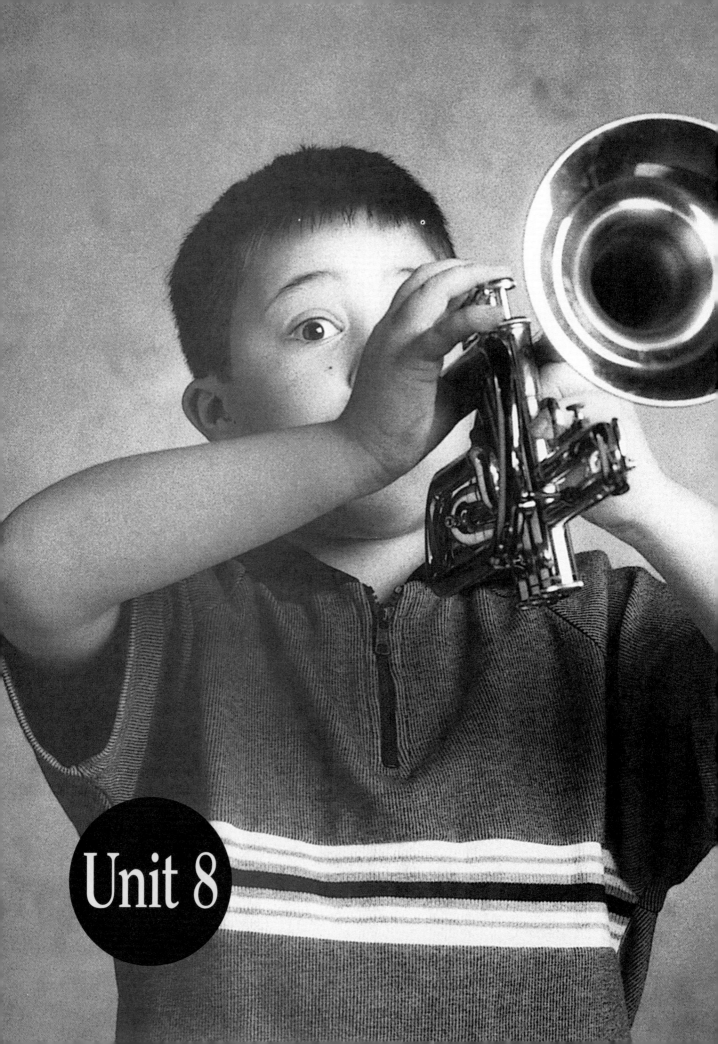

Unit 8

Consumer and Community Health

Before You Buy

Vocabulary

health product: an item that is used for physical, mental, or social health.

health service: a person or place that helps improve your physical, mental, or social health.

advertising: a form of selling products and services.

appeal: a statement used to get consumers to buy a product or service.

media: ways of sending messages to consumers.

media literacy: being able to see and evaluate the messages you get from the media.

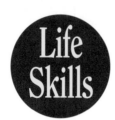

Life Skills

- **I will check out sources of health information.**
- **I will check ways technology, media, and culture influence health choices.**
- **I will choose safe and healthful products.**

A **health product** is an item that is used for physical, mental, or social health. You make decisions about which health products you will use. For example, you might like a certain shampoo more than another one. Perhaps you like it because of how your hair feels after you use it. Maybe you think it smells good. Perhaps you buy it because it is cheap. You need to choose health products wisely. You need to learn how advertising influences your choices.

The Lesson Objectives

- Discuss ways to make wise choices about health products and services.
- Discuss ad appeals that try to influence your choices.
- Tell why you need to have media literacy.
- Discuss kinds of technology you can use to learn about health.
- Tell how to check your sources of health information.

How Can I Make Wise Choices About Health Products and Services?

Your family spends part of its income on health products and services. A health product is an item that is used for physical, mental, or social health. Shampoo, soap, and toothpaste are health products. A **health service** is a person or place that helps improve your physical, mental, or social health. A doctor or dentist provides health services. A clinic or hospital provides health services. You can make wise choices about health products and services.

Know why you are buying a health product or service. You might think you need something until you ask yourself whether you can live without it. Ask yourself why you are spending money on a product or service. Ask yourself if you really need the product or service.

Get facts and read product labels. Try to learn as much as you can about a product or service before you buy it. Look at magazines that contain research on products and services. Learn about the contents of a product by reading the label. Product labels list the name and address of the company that make the product. You can write to the company if you have a question.

Find out who recommends the service or product. You might ask your doctor, pharmacist, and dentist for advice. Agencies such as the American Cancer Society might recommend a product or service. Sometimes, there is a seal of approval on a product label. For example, some toothpaste labels state that the product is accepted by the American Dental Association.

Compare the price. Similar products and services might have different prices. For example, a pharmacy might have its own brand of aspirin. It might cost less than a brand of aspirin that is shown on TV.

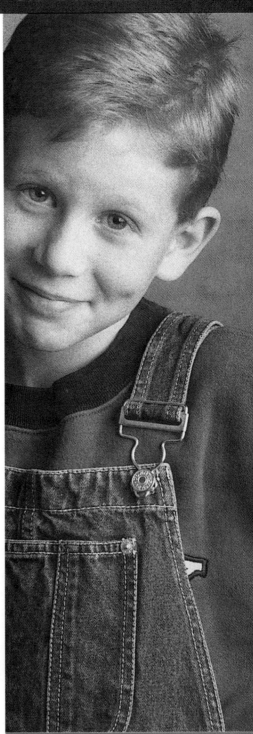

What Ad Appeals Try to Influence My Choices?

Advertising is a form of selling products and services. An *advertisement* or *ad* is a paid announcement. A *commercial* is an ad on television or radio. Look closely at ads and commercials. People who write ads and commercials use appeals. An **appeal** is a statement used to get consumers to buy a product or service. Knowing about the following appeals might help you decide whether you need a product or service.

"You'll be popular if you own this product." Wrong! People are popular because they are friendly and considerate. People do not become popular because of the clothes they wear or the things they own. Work on being friendly and considerate if you want to be popular.

"I'm famous. You'll be just like me if you own this product." Wrong again. You might admire a famous person because of his or her talent or skills. You might want to be like this person. Practice your skills and develop your talents. Purchasing a product will not make you become like the famous person. Remember, famous people are paid to advertise products. They might not even use the products themselves!

"If you buy Product A, you can have Product B for free!" So what? Ask yourself whether you really need Product A or Product B. Chances are, you can do without either product.

"Everyone else has one, so you should have one, too." A *fad* is a style or product that is popular for a short time. When "everyone" has something simply because it is in style, it probably is a fad. Again, ask yourself whether you really need the product.

Get the Facts!

Ads often leave out facts that might make you not want to buy the products. For example, cigarette ads do not mention that smoking harms health. The required health warning appears in small print. Think about what facts advertisers leave out.

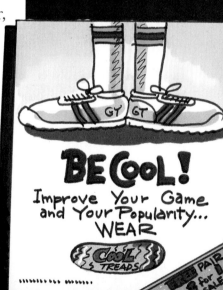

BE COOL!
Improve Your Game and Your Popularity... WEAR Cool Treads

Why Do I Need to Have Media Literacy?

Media are ways of sending messages to consumers. Some kinds of media are television, radio, magazines, newspapers, books, and the Internet. Suppose you watch a news report, read a magazine ad, or see a billboard. You get messages from the media. **Media literacy** is being able to see and evaluate the messages you get from the media.

You need to have media literacy:

- To notice messages in the media.
- To notice the appeals that are used in messages.
- To react to media messages in a responsible way.

Media Literacy Buff

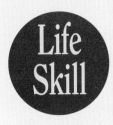

Life Skill

I will check ways technology, media, and culture influence health choices.

Materials: Magazine ad, paper, pen or pencil

Directions: Be a media literacy buff. See and respond responsibly to the messages in media.

Activity

1. **Find a magazine ad that is meant to get someone your age to buy a product.** The product might be a CD, a piece of clothing, a snack food, or a beverage.

2. **Answer these questions.**
   - Who wrote the ad?
   - How do I know the ad is for someone my age?
   - What is the ad trying to get me to do?
   - Is the ad trying to get me to do something responsible? (Think about the *Guidelines for Making Responsible Decisions™.*)
   - Did the person who wrote the ad leave out any facts? Why?

What Kinds of Technology Help Me Learn About Health?

You probably use technology every day. You watch television programs. You listen to music, ads, and programs on the radio. At school, you might use a computer. Your family might have a computer. Technology is a way to learn about health.

Television programs

There are many television programs that focus on health. Some of the programs are specials. There might be a special on HIV and AIDS or one on heart disease. Some talk shows include interviews with health experts. The local and national news might have facts about health.

CD-ROMs

A *CD-ROM* (SEE·DEE·RAHM) is a computer disc that stores computer programs. There might be text, pictures, music, and movies. These can contain facts about health. They can contain games you can play to learn about health. They might contain programs to test your health knowledge. They might allow you to check your habits. You need a computer with a CD-ROM drive to use a CD-ROM.

The World Wide Web

The *World Wide Web,* or Web, is a computer system that lets you find information, pictures, and text. You can find information about most health topics on the Web. Many health agencies have Web sites. A *Web site* is a collection of files or "pages" kept on a computer. You need a computer, a modem, and a special computer account to use the Web. Most libraries have these for your use.

Caution:

Anyone can place information on the Web. This means that you must carefully judge the worth of any information you find on the Web. Whenever you find health information, use the questions in the box to the right to check the information.

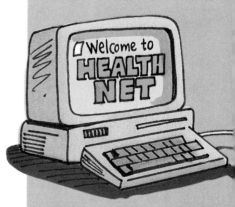

Use these questions to evaluate the worth of health information.

What is the source of the information? You can depend on health information from government agencies, community organizations, and professional organizations. You should not depend on health information from sources that are not connected to one of these groups.

Is the information based on scientific research? The information should not be someone's opinion. You should be able to get copies of the research.

Does your doctor or dentist believe the information? You can ask your doctor or dentist when you have doubts about health information.

Can you get more information if you request it? Other sources should have similar information.

Some Health Organizations That Have Web Sites

American Medical Association

Centers for Disease Control and Prevention (CDC)

American Cancer Society

American Heart Association

American Red Cross

Food and Drug Administration

Environmental Protection Agency

Lesson 33

Review

Health Content

Write answers to the following:

1. What are four ways you can make wise choices about health products and services? **page 253**
2. What are four ad appeals that try to influence your choices? **page 254**
3. Why do you need to have media literacy? **page 255**
4. What are three kinds of technology you can use to learn about health? **page 256**
5. What questions can you use to check your sources of health information? **page 257**

Vocabulary

Write a separate sentence using each of the vocabulary words listed on page 252.

Quality Control

Vocabulary

time management plan: a plan that shows how a person will spend time.

consumer: a person who judges information and buys products and services.

budget: a plan for spending and saving money.

income: the money a person receives or earns.

expenses: products and services a person needs to buy.

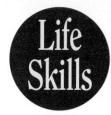

- I will spend time and money wisely.
- I will choose healthful entertainment.

You have homework, chores, and school activities. You want to spend time with your friends. You want to spend time with your family. You need to make sure your life is balanced. A balanced life includes time for yourself, time for your chores and homework, time for exercise, and time with family and friends. You need to plan time for all these things. A balanced life also means you spend your money wisely and choose healthful TV programs.

The Lesson Objectives

- Tell how to make a plan to manage your time.
- Tell how to make a budget.
- Tell how too much TV can affect your health.
- Discuss five characteristics of healthful TV programs.

How Can I Make a Plan to Manage Time?

You probably have many activities you enjoy. How do you make time for them all? Try making a time management plan. A **time management plan** is a plan that shows how a person will spend time. You can write a time management plan in hourly time blocks. Begin by writing down the time that you wake up in the morning. Then, write in everything you must do that already has a set time. For example, you know what hours you will be in school. If you are on a soccer team or in another school activity, you know what times you are expected to be there. If you have a paper route, you know what times you must deliver papers. Include family activities that have set times.

Next, make a list of things you do that do not have exact times. For example, you will need time to do your homework. You will need time to do your chores. Plan times to bathe, wash your hair, brush and floss your teeth, sleep, and eat healthful snacks. Write these on your time management plan.

Think of other activities that are good for your health. Plan a time for exercise. Plan a time to read and work puzzles. Plan to spend time with your family and friends. Be sure that you plan time to be alone.

Keep a list of homework and other things you need to do. Write each new task on your list. Write when you must complete it. Cross off each task when you have finished it. You will always know what you have to do. You will not forget to do homework or chores. You will save time for activities you enjoy.

Keep Your Desk Neat!

You can save time at school by keeping your desk neat and tidy. Do not just stuff things in your desk until it overflows. Keep your papers in folders. Keep your supplies in order. You will be able to find things quickly.

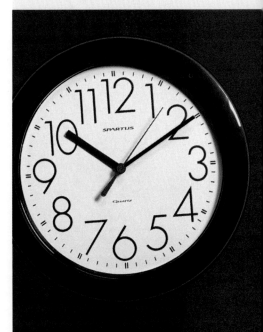

Follow a...
Health Behavior Contract

Copy the health behavior contract on a separate sheet of paper.

DO NOT WRITE IN THIS BOOK.

Name: _____ **Date:** _____

Life Skill: I will spend time and money wisely.

Effect on My Health: When my desk is neat, I will be able to find things easily. I will not waste time looking for things. I will not lose important projects or papers. My papers will not be crushed because they were stuffed in my desk. I will be able to find all my supplies. I will not be stressed because I cannot find papers or supplies.

My Plan: I will clean out my desk. I will put my papers in folders or notebooks. I will keep my supplies in order. I will throw away anything I no longer need. Then, I will straighten up my desk at the end of each day. If I take a few minutes each day to tidy up, my desk will not become messy again. I will make a mark on my calendar each day that I clean up my desk before leaving.

My Calendar	M	T	W	Th	F	S	S

How My Plan Worked: I kept my desk neat and clean. I was able to find papers and supplies quickly and easily. I did not waste time looking for things. My papers were not crushed.

How Can I Make a Budget?

You and your family are consumers. A **consumer** is a person who judges information and buys products and services. You should be a responsible consumer. You should learn how to make a budget for your money. A **budget** is a plan for spending and saving money.

List your income when you make your budget. **Income** is the money a person receives or earns. You might get an allowance from your parents. You might earn money if you childsit or mow lawns. Your relatives might give you money for a special occasion, such as your birthday.

You will want to save part of your income. You might want to save to buy something special, such as a bike. You might want to save money to go to college. Learning to save is an important part of making a budget.

You also will need to list your expenses on your budget. **Expenses** are products and services a person needs to buy. You might pay for your ticket to go to the movies. You might buy a new book or pay for your haircut. You might buy presents for family and friends. You might give part of your income to help with family expenses.

Talk about your budget with your parents or guardian. They want you to know how to manage money. They want you to spend money wisely. They want you to learn to save. These are skills you need now. These are skills you will need as an adult. When you have these skills, you are responsible.

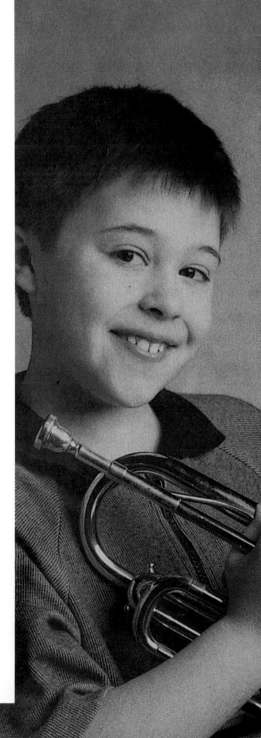

How Can I Decide What TV Programs to Watch?

How much TV do you watch? Many children watch more than four hours of TV each day. There are reasons to limit the number of hours you watch TV. There are reasons to choose TV programs carefully.

Research shows interesting facts about the effects of watching TV.

Watching too much TV can affect your imagination.

You use your imagination to write a story. You use it to paint a picture. Suppose you watch a lot of TV. You are less likely to be involved in activities where you use your imagination.

Watching too much TV can affect your behavior.

There is too much violence on TV. Children who watch violence might copy wrong behaviors. They might think wrong behaviors are okay.

Watching too much TV limits your time for physical activity.

Children who spend four hours watching TV do not have time for physical activity. They are less fit than other children.

Watching too much TV can affect study habits.

TV programs usually have breaks for ads every seven minutes. Suppose you get used to seven minute breaks. Your attention span will be short. It will be hard for you to concentrate for more than seven minutes. This can affect schoolwork. It will be hard for you to listen or do homework.

Make Top-Notch TV Choices

- Plan ahead what shows you will watch.
- Do not watch TV until your homework is done.
- Plan with your parents or guardian what shows you can watch.
- Make a list of other activities that you can do instead of watching TV. Then do them!

Guidelines for Choosing TV Programs

1. TV programs should be approved for your age group.
2. TV programs should be approved by your parents or guardian.
3. TV programs should not present harmful drug use as acceptable behavior.
4. TV programs should not present violence as acceptable behavior.
5. TV programs should not present sex outside of marriage as responsible behavior.

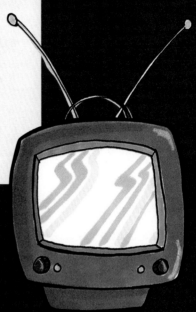

Lesson 34

Review

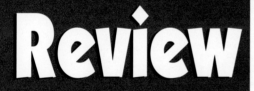

Vocabulary

Write a separate sentence using each of the vocabulary words listed on page 258.

Health Content

Write answers to the following:

1. How can you make a plan to manage your time? **page 259**
2. How can you keep from forgetting homework or chores? **page 259**
3. How can you make a budget? **page 261**
4. How can too much TV affect your health? **page 262**
5. What are five guidelines for choosing healthful TV programs? **page 263**

Consumer Support

Vocabulary

quackery: a method of selling worthless products and services.

Better Business Bureau (BBB): a group that encourages businesses to treat customers fairly.

Food and Drug Administration (FDA): a federal agency that checks the safety and effectiveness of drugs and medical devices.

Federal Trade Commission (FTC): a federal agency that deals with false advertising.

volunteer: a person who provides a service without being paid.

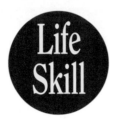

Life Skill

- **I will cooperate with community and school health helpers.**

As a consumer, you need to know the difference between true medical advice and quackery. Medical advice is supported by research. It comes from doctors, nurses, and groups such as the American Medical Association. **Quackery** (KWA·kuh·ree) is a method of selling worthless products and services. You can protect yourself against quackery.

The Lesson Objectives

- Discuss groups that protect consumers.
- Explain what you can do if you are not satisfied with a product or service.
- Explain ways you can volunteer.

What Groups Protect Consumers?

Where might you get help if you or your parent or guardian think you have been a victim of quackery? Where might you get help if you have heard an ad that makes false claims? A *false claim* is a statement that is not true. Where can you get help if you get false information or products that do not work through the mail? Many consumer groups can help.

The **Better Business Bureau (BBB)** is a group that encourages businesses to treat customers fairly. People might call the BBB before they make a purchase. The BBB has a list with the names of many companies. They keep a file of complaints that have been made about a company's products or services. You can call the BBB if you have a complaint or question about a company's record of service.

The **Food and Drug Administration (FDA)** is a federal agency that checks the safety and effectiveness of drugs and medical devices. The FDA checks food and cosmetics. The FDA makes sure that foods and products are labeled correctly. The FDA also checks OTC drugs to see that the directions for use are safe and correct. If there is a problem with a health product you use, you can contact the FDA.

The **Federal Trade Commission (FTC)** is a federal agency that deals with false advertising. Anything that is printed or said on radio or TV about foods, drugs, and cosmetics should be true. If you are aware of false advertising, contact the FTC.

The United States Postal Service works to protect you from being tricked by products, services, or devices sold through the mail. You can contact your local post office if you think you have been tricked by something you received in the mail.

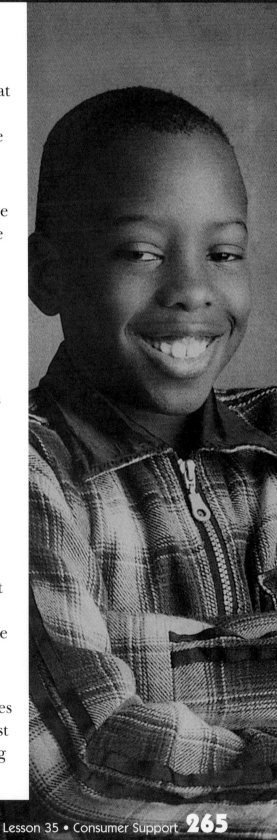

What Can I Do If I Am Not Satisfied with a Product or Service?

You need to act if a product or service is not what it was promised to be. You might decide with your parents or guardian to make a consumer complaint. A *consumer complaint* is a way of telling others that you are not happy with a product or service.

To make a consumer complaint, you need to have the product and the sales receipt. You should contact the person who sold you the product or service. There are three ways to do this.

- You can set a time to talk to this person.
- You can call the person by telephone.
- You can write a letter.

Always keep copies of any letters you write. Always be polite. Include the following when you make a complaint:

- A description of the product or service
- The complete address of the place where you or your parents or guardian bought the product or service
- The date the product or service was bought
- How you paid for the product or service
- The reason you are not satisfied
- The result you want; for example, do you want your money back? Do you want the product replaced?

Suppose you write a letter to make a consumer complaint, and no one responds. Contact a manager or the company that made the product. Provide the same information you provided in your letter. Suppose you still get no response. Contact one of the agencies listed on page 265.

When You Purchase Products

- Keep your sales receipts. Ask your parents or guardian where to keep them. Keep them even after you have used the product.

- Keep all of the packaging that comes with the product. Some companies will not take returns unless you have it.

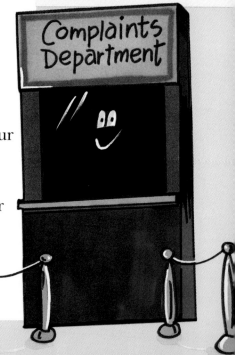

What Are Ways I Can Volunteer?

Do you want to build your self-respect? Perhaps you would like to meet new people. Maybe you would like to learn a new skill. You can gain all these benefits by being a volunteer. A **volunteer** is a person who offers a service without being paid. Being a volunteer can improve your health. You feel good about yourself because you are helping others. You boost your immune system because you feel good about yourself. You might become ill less often. There are many ways you can be a volunteer.

Look for things your community needs. Is a local food pantry short on food? A food pantry is a place where food is collected and then given to people who need it. You can collect canned food to give to the food pantry. Does a local park have a lot of litter on the ground? Ask your parents or guardian to help you form a group to clean up the litter. Does your community have a recycling program? If not, start one. Are there people in your community who need clothing? Start a clothing drive to collect clothing to give to people who need it. You might see a problem and think, "Someone should do something about that." YOU are someone. YOU can solve problems. Don't wait for other people to solve all the problems you see. You can make a difference.

Think about activities you enjoy. Do you like to act or sing? You could form a group to perform a play or music program for younger children or older adults. Do you enjoy sports like swimming or running? You could participate in events to raise money to help others. Are you very good at a school subject? You could tutor a younger student who needs help with that subject.

Healthy Helper Syndrome

Suppose you agree to volunteer. Did you know that being a volunteer can improve health? Health experts have studied the healthy helper syndrome. They believe positive changes take place inside your body when you volunteer to help others. So, help others and help yourself at the same time!

Get permission from your parents or guardian to call a local nursing home. Ask if you can visit a resident who receives few visitors. Visit the person regularly. You can keep him or her from feeling lonely. Older adults often have many stories and memories to share with you. Ask the person to tell you about special events and other memories he or she has. Bring pictures, projects, or other items to share with him or her. Bring board games to play. You might offer to help the person write letters to friends and family members. You might read books out loud, or make a tape of yourself reading to give to the person. Be sure the person is allowed to eat any food you bring before you give it to him or her. Always visit when you say you will.

Make cards for people who are in the hospital. Learn first aid, so you can help when others are ill or injured. The American Red Cross offers courses in first aid. Help an older adult weed his or her garden or do odd jobs around the house. How many other ideas can you think of?

Sometimes, an area has a natural disaster such as a tornado or flood. People in the area might lose their homes and belongings. You can help by sending food or clothing. Suppose a natural disaster occurs nearby. You might be able to help by serving food or cleaning up safe areas. Ask your parents or guardian what you can do to help victims of a natural disaster.

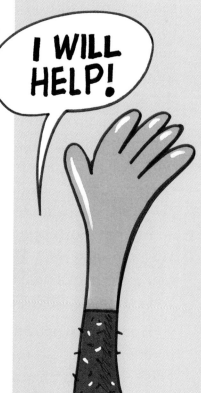

Check out volunteer organizations in your community. Ask your parents or guardian and your teacher to suggest places where you could volunteer. Remember, people count on you when you agree to volunteer. Show up on time if you promise you will be somewhere. Do your work with a smile. Call right away if you are ill or if you know you will be late.

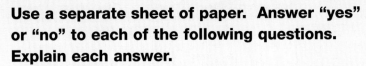

Use... Guidelines for Making Responsible Decisions™

You buy a radio. You accidentally break it after you have had it for a week. Your classmate suggests that you take the radio back to the store. She suggests you say the radio was broken when you bought it.

?

Use a separate sheet of paper. Answer "yes" or "no" to each of the following questions. Explain each answer.

1. Is it healthful to say the radio was broken when you bought it?

2. Is it safe to say the radio was broken when you bought it?

3. Do you follow rules and laws if you say the radio was broken when you bought it?

4. Do you show respect for yourself and others if you say the radio was broken when you bought it?

5. Do you follow your family's guidelines if you say the radio was broken when you bought it?

6. Do you show good character if you say the radio was broken when you bought it?

What is the responsible decision to make?

Lesson 35

Review ◆

Vocabulary

Write a separate sentence using each of the vocabulary words listed on page 264.

Health Content

Write answers to the following:

1. What are four groups that protect consumers? **page 265**

2. What can you do if you are not satisfied with a product or service? **page 266**

3. What should you include in a consumer complaint? **page 266**

4. How can being a volunteer improve your health? **page 267**

5. What are at least five ways you can be a volunteer? **pages 267–268**

Three Cheers for Health Careers

Vocabulary

career: the work that a person prepares for and does through life.

health career: a job in the health field for which one trains.

shadowing: spending time with a mentor as he or she performs work activities.

mentor: a responsible person who helps a younger person.

certificate: a document issued by a nongovernment agency that states a person is qualified to perform a certain job.

license: a document issued by a government agency that states a person can legally perform a certain job.

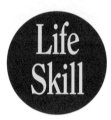

Life Skill

● **I will learn about health careers.**

Do you know what you want to be when you grow up? You might want to consider a health career. A **career** is the work that a person prepares for and does through life. A **health career** is a job in the health field for which one trains. There are many health careers you might choose. Begin now to learn about health careers.

The Lesson Objectives

● Discuss how you can learn about health careers.
● Describe health careers you might choose.

How Can I Learn About Health Careers?

You might think that a person with a health career must work in a hospital. This is not true. Your health teacher has a health career. So does a police officer and a firefighter. These people help protect the health and safety of others.

There are several ways you can learn about health careers. You can check out books from the library on different health careers. You can search the World Wide Web for information on health careers. Remember to use the questions on pages 256–257 to check any information you find on the Web.

You might talk to people who have different health careers. Get permission from your parents or guardian to call a person who has a health career that interests you. Ask if you can meet with that person to talk about his or her career. Many professionals are happy to talk to young people about their work. Ask questions about tasks the person performs, the education the person has, and what the person likes and dislikes about his or her job.

Ask your parents or guardian and your teacher about shadowing someone who has a health career. **Shadowing** is spending time with a mentor as he or she performs work activities. A **mentor** is a responsible person who helps a younger person. A mentor can help you learn what you would like to do as a career. When you shadow a person who has a health career, you watch what the person does in his or her job. You learn the responsibilities the person has. You are able to see whether you would enjoy having the health career.

Keep a Journal If You Shadow

Suppose you shadow someone. Take a notepad with you so that you can keep a journal. The person you shadow might get very busy. Jot down questions to ask later. Write down tasks a mentor performs that are of interest to you.

What Health Careers Might I Choose?

Most health careers require some kind of special training. Some require you to go to college. Some require you to go to graduate school or medical school for an advanced degree. Some careers might require a certificate or license. A **certificate** is a document issued by a nongovernment agency that states a person is qualified to perform a certain job. A **license** is a document issued by a government agency that states a person can legally perform a certain job.

Some health careers you might choose appear on the next two pages. Perhaps you will see several that interest you. If so, think about talking to people who have those health careers. You might be able to shadow those people. Write down information you learn from these people. You can look back at it when choosing careers about which you want to learn more.

There is something you should know about health careers. The number of senior citizens continues to increase. This has created more jobs in health careers involving senior citizens. You might want to volunteer to work with the older population. Then you will know if this type of health career suits you.

The number of health careers in technology continues to increase, too. Suppose you like working on a computer. Perhaps you like to find information on the Web. A health career in technology might be for you.

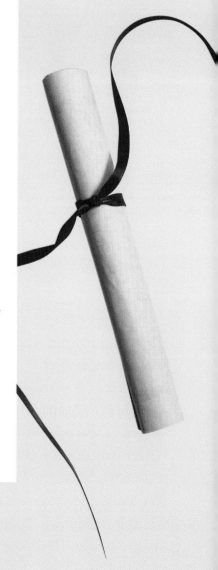

Health Education Teacher

A *health education teacher* is a teacher who helps students develop health knowledge, practice life skills, and form healthful habits. Health education teachers need teaching skills. They need knowledge of health information. Health education teachers have college degrees and knowledge of health. They have teaching certificates from a government agency. Health education teachers work in public and private schools.

Emergency Medical Technician (EMT)

An *emergency medical technician* (tek·NI·shuhn) *(EMT)* is a person who takes care of people in emergency situations before they reach the hospital. EMTs perform first aid, help stop bleeding, and treat injuries. They perform rescue breathing and CPR. EMTs take patients to the hospital in ambulances. EMTs have high school diplomas and special EMT training. They have certificates. EMTs work in hospitals and ambulances.

Physician

A *physician* is a medical doctor who is trained to diagnose and treat illnesses. Physicians examine patients. They diagnose and treat illnesses and injuries. Some physicians practice general medicine. These physicians take care of their patients' whole bodies. Other physicians are specialists. A specialist is a physician who has additional training in a particular area. One kind of specialist is a podiatrist, who treats problems with feet. Physicians have college degrees and degrees from medical schools. They have training in hospitals or medical offices. They have certificates and licenses. Physicians work in hospitals, clinics, and private practices.

School Nurse

A *school nurse* is a nurse who works in a school and takes care of ill or injured students and teachers. School nurses have knowledge of health care, nutrition, and other health topics. School nurses have degrees in nursing. They have licenses and certificates. They work in public and private schools.

Dietitian

A *dietitian* is a nutrition expert. Dietitians help people learn about healthful diets. They plan healthful menus for schools, hospitals, and other institutions. They help people learn to plan healthful meals for themselves and their families. They know how to develop menus and prepare food. Dietitians have college degrees. They have knowledge of nutrition, chemistry, biology, and physiology. They have licenses. Dietitians work in schools, restaurants, hotels, hospitals, nursing homes, and company cafeterias. They also work with individual patients.

School Psychologist

A *psychologist* (sy·KAH·luh·jist) is a person who applies knowledge about the mind and ways people behave to help people solve problems. A *school psychologist* is a psychologist who is trained to work with students, teachers, and parents and guardians. School psychologists help students solve problems they might have. They help resolve conflicts. They help teachers, parents, and guardians decide what school subjects students are ready to learn. School psychologists have master's or doctoral degrees. They have licenses. They work in schools.

Optometrist

An *optometrist* (ahp·TAH·muh·trist) is a person who is trained to examine eyes and diagnose and treat vision and eye problems. They use special equipment to diagnose vision problems. They prescribe eyeglasses and contact lenses. Optometrists have degrees from schools of optometry.

Dental Hygienist

A *dental hygienist* (DEN·tuhl hy·JE·nist) is a person who works with a dentist to take care of patients' teeth. Dental hygienists clean teeth and take X-rays. They apply fluorides and sealants to help prevent cavities. Dental hygienists have college degrees. They have licenses. They work in dentists' offices and schools.

Guidance Counselor

A *guidance counselor* is a person who helps students solve problems, plan school subjects, and learn about careers. Guidance counselors listen to students' problems. They help students make plans to solve problems. They help students explore career possibilities. Guidance counselors have college degrees. They might have master's degrees. They have certificates. Guidance counselors work in schools.

Career Tryouts

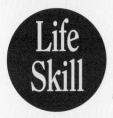

Life Skill I will learn about health careers.

Materials: None

Directions: Follow the steps to create a cheer for a health career.

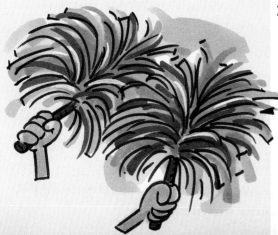

1. **Choose one of the health careers described in this lesson.** Reread the description of the health career.

2. **Create a cheer for the health career you chose.** Your cheer should include information about the career. For example, you might begin by saying, "I am (your name). I am here to try out for a health career!"

3. **Perform your cheer for your class.**

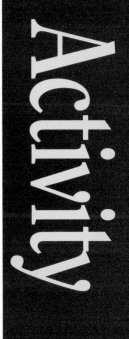

Activity

Lesson 36

Review

Vocabulary

Write a separate sentence using each of the vocabulary words listed on page 270.

Health Content

Write answers to the following:

1. What are ways you can learn about health careers? **page 271**

2. What is the difference between a certificate and a license? **page 272**

3. What are nine health careers you might choose? **pages 273–274**

4. What education do EMTs have? **page 273**

5. What does a dietitian do? **page 274**

Unit 8 Review

Health Content

Review your answers for each Lesson Review in this unit. Write answers to the following questions.

1. What are four ways ad appeals try to influence your choices about products or services? **Lesson 33 page 254**

2. What are four questions you can use to evaluate sources of health information? **Lesson 33 page 257**

3. How might you develop a plan to manage your time? **Lesson 34 page 259**

4. In what ways can watching too much TV harm your health? **Lesson 34 page 262**

5. What are five ways you can tell whether a TV program is healthful? **Lesson 34 page 263**

6. What action can you take if you are not satisfied with a product or service? **Lesson 35 page 266**

7. What are ways being a volunteer can improve your health? **Lesson 35 page 267**

8. How can you learn about health careers? **Lesson 36 page 271**

9. How can a mentor help you? **Lesson 36 page 271**

10. What tasks does a dental hygienist perform? **Lesson 36 page 274**

Guidelines for Making Responsible Decisions™

You see an ad for a vitamin that promises to make you strong, healthy, and attractive. You are tempted to order the vitamin. Use a separate sheet of paper. Answer "yes" or "no" to each of the following questions. Explain each answer.

1. Is it healthful to order the vitamin?
2. Is it safe to order the vitamin?
3. Do you follow rules and laws if you order the vitamin?
4. Do you show respect for yourself and others if you order the vitamin?
5. Do you follow your family's guidelines if you order the vitamin?
6. Do you show good character if you order the vitamin?

What is the responsible decision to make?

Multicultural Health

Find a magazine from another country. Look closely at the ads. How are they the same as ads in this country? How are they different?

Vocabulary

Number a sheet of paper from 1–10. Read each definition. Next to each number on your sheet of paper, write the vocabulary word that matches the definition.

health product	quackery
advertising	volunteer
media literacy	mentor
consumer	certificate
budget	career

1. A person who provides a service without being paid. **Lesson 35**

2. A plan for saving and spending money. **Lesson 34**

3. A document issued by a nongovernment agency that states a person is qualified to perform a certain job. **Lesson 36**

4. A form of selling products and services. **Lesson 33**

5. Being able to see and evaluate the messages you get from the media. **Lesson 33**

6. A person who judges information and buys products and services. **Lesson 34**

7. The work that a person prepares for and does through life. **Lesson 36**

8. A method of selling worthless products and services. **Lesson 35**

9. An item that is used for physical, mental, or social health. **Lesson 33**

10. A responsible person who helps a younger person. **Lesson 36**

Health Literacy

Effective Communication

Make a pamphlet that describes how to evaluate ads. Share the pamphlet with a younger student.

Self-Directed Learning

Find out about a health career not described in this lesson. Write three paragraphs about the health career you chose.

Critical Thinking

Why is it important to choose safe and healthful products?

Responsible Citizenship

Make a list of Web sites that provide reliable health information. Share the list with your classmates.

Family Involvement

Discuss the information on pages 262–263 with your parents or guardian. Make a plan for viewing healthful TV programs with your family.

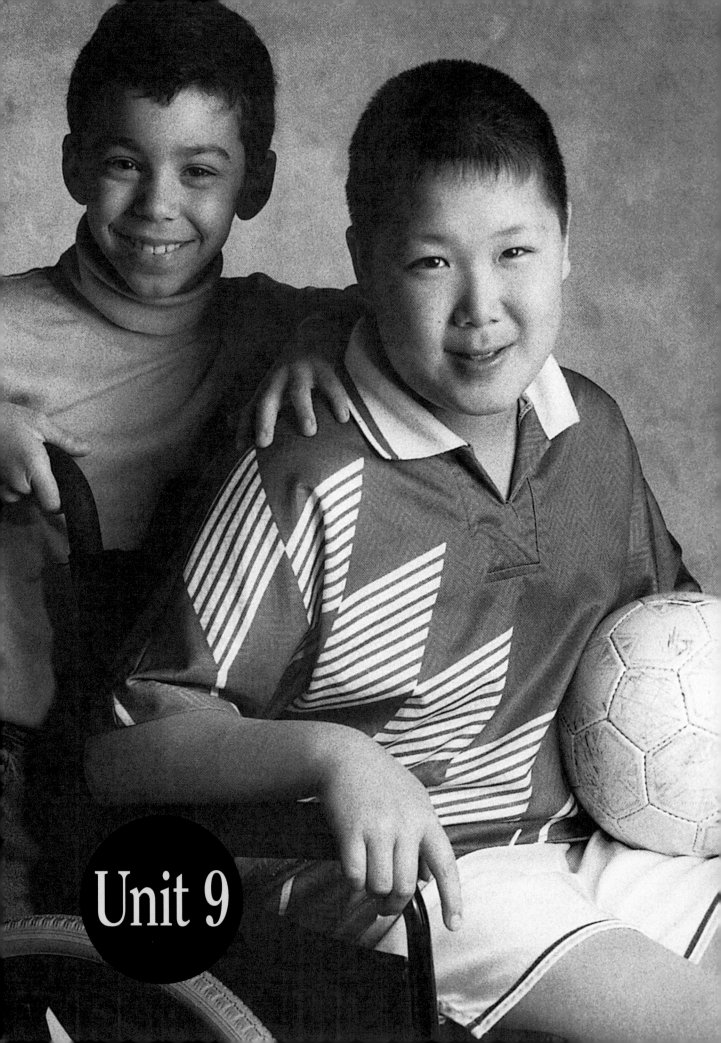

Unit 9

Environmental Health

Pollution Solution

Vocabulary

environment: everything that is around you.

pollution: the presence of substances in the environment that can harm your health.

acid rain: rainfall that includes pollutants.

radon: a radioactive gas that you cannot see or smell.

toxic waste: waste that is poisonous.

water-treatment plant: a place where water from nearby rivers and streams is made safe to drink.

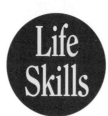
Life Skills

- **I will help protect my environment.**
- **I will keep the air, water, and land clean and safe.**

The **environment** is everything that is around you. Every day, you experience the environment. Every day, you breathe air, drink water, and walk on land. Did you know there might be pollutants in the air you breathe and the water you drink? A *pollutant* is something that has a harmful effect on the environment. You can help lower the amount of pollutants that are released into the environment.

The Lesson Objectives

- Explain how air pollution affects your health.
- Discuss ways you can help reduce air pollution.
- Explain how water pollution affects your health.
- Discuss ways you can help reduce water pollution.
- Explain how land pollution affects your health.
- Discuss ways you can help reduce land pollution.

How Does Air Pollution Affect My Health?

You need air to stay alive. You need clean air to stay healthy. Sometimes, the air you breathe is filled with pollution. **Pollution** (puh·LOO·shuhn) is the presence of substances in the environment that can harm your health. Air pollution results when fuels such as oil, coal, and gasoline are burned, and harmful wastes enter the air. These wastes include fumes, dust, and dirt. These wastes remain in the air and are inhaled by people. Polluted air can harm parts of your body such as your throat, lungs, and eyes.

Carbon monoxide is a harmful gas found in polluted air. *Carbon monoxide* (KAR·buhn muh·NAHK·SYD) is an odorless, colorless, poisonous gas. This gas comes from burning fuels and also is found in cigarette smoke. Breathing this gas causes people to get headaches and feel tired.

Burning coal and oil produces smoke and gases that pollute the air. This air pollution can cause acid rain. **Acid rain** is rainfall that includes pollutants. Acid rain can harm the water in a lake, fish, and cause plants to die. Over several years, acid rain can cause concrete and stone in buildings and statues to wear away.

There is also indoor air pollution. One type of indoor air pollution is cigarette smoke. Smoke gets into the air when someone who smokes exhales. This smoke is inhaled by everyone in a room.

Another pollutant that is found indoors is radon. **Radon** (RAY·dahn) is a radioactive gas that you cannot see or smell. Radon enters a building through cracks in basement floors and walls and becomes trapped in the building. Radon is dangerous because it can cause lung cancer.

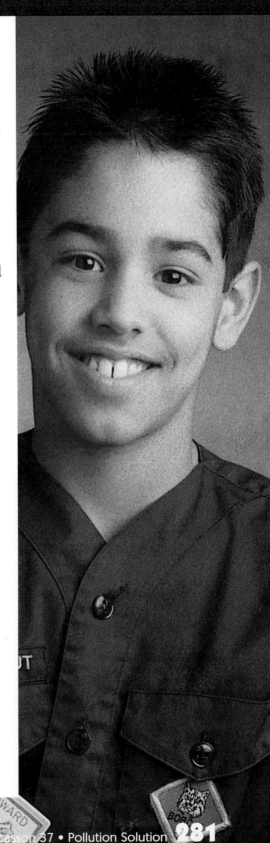

How Can I Help Reduce Air Pollution?

One major cause of air pollution is car exhaust. Exhaust is a gas waste produced by fuels that have been burned. The EPA has made rules to control these and other wastes. The *Environmental Protection Agency (EPA)* is a government office that makes rules and enforces laws to help control pollution.

The EPA requires that parts be put on cars to filter wastes from car exhaust. Because of EPA rules, the amount of harmful wastes that enter the air from cars has been lowered. All harmful wastes from car exhaust have not yet been totally controlled.

You know that radon is one type of indoor pollutant. Radon is radioactive gas that you cannot see or smell. Radon enters a basement from cracks in the basement floors and walls. You can get a test kit to see if radon is in your home. If you find radon, take steps to lower your family's risk of disease from radon. One way to lower radon levels is to increase air flow in the home. You can use fans to help move this gas out through windows or doors.

Many agencies are helping to tell people about the dangers of air pollution. Two of these health agencies are the American Lung Association and the American Cancer Society. Because of them, people are working to reduce indoor pollution. Many people do not allow smoking in their homes. Many businesses do not allow smoking in their buildings. Most airlines do not allow smoking on their planes. In the United States, there is no smoking on airline flights shorter than two hours. Airlines must have a smoke-free area on longer flights.

Ways You Can Help Lower Air Pollution

- Walk or ride your bike to nearby places instead of having a parent or guardian drive you.
- Do not smoke. Have a no-smoking policy in your home. Ask other people not to smoke around you.
- Plant trees. Trees help filter some gases in the atmosphere. They make oxygen. House plants might help reduce some indoor air pollution.
- Make sure you have plenty of airflow when you use chemicals such as hobby glues. The fumes can be harmful.
- Do not burn trash or yard waste.

How Does Water Pollution Affect My Health?

Water makes up over half of your weight. Every cell in your body needs it. Without water, a person can live only a few days.

You can get water from many places. The water in your home might come from a lake, river, or well. Clean water is important for good health.

Fish live in rivers, lakes, and oceans. Fish are a source of healthful food. It is important that fish come from clean water so that they are free from harmful substances.

Sometimes, water becomes polluted. There are different ways this can happen. Sewage might be dumped into a water supply. *Sewage* is waste material carried off by sewers. Sewage includes human and chemical waste material.

Toxic waste is waste that is poisonous. Toxic waste can harm the environment. For example, some industries might dump chemicals into large bodies of water. If this water is not treated, these toxic wastes can enter a water supply. People who drink this water might become sick.

Toxic waste can pollute water in other ways. Suppose harmful chemicals are used to grow food or kill weeds or insects. The chemicals might get into the ground. During a heavy rain, the chemicals might run off the land and pollute a lake or river. They might also pollute water in wells.

People throw away toxic waste in heavy containers buried under the ground. But if these containers leak, the waste can enter water that we drink. Toxic waste is dangerous. The waste can cause cancer and many other diseases.

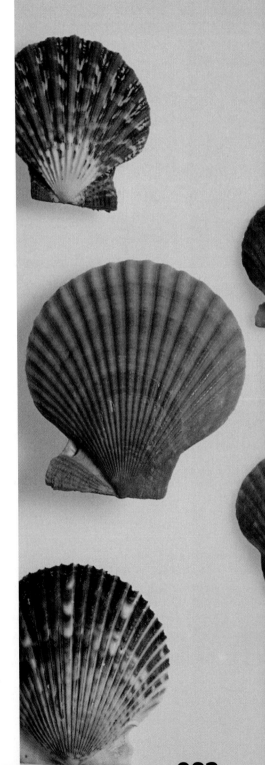

How Can I Help Reduce Water Pollution?

Dumping wastes into water causes water pollution. Many factories are located near water. Many kinds of chemicals are used to make products. As these chemicals are used, wastes are produced. For many years, factory wastes were dumped into nearby rivers and streams. This polluted the water. As rivers and streams flowed into oceans, the oceans also became polluted.

Today, there are laws to control water pollution. These laws require factories to filter and collect wastes. Factories are not allowed to dump wastes or use certain chemicals to make products. Some chemicals harm life in the water. Through these efforts to control water pollution, many rivers and streams are kept clean.

However, many chemicals run off the land into the water. Some farmers put chemicals on their crops. Some people put chemicals on their lawns. When it rains, the rain can wash the chemicals into water.

Most communities have water-treatment plants. A **water-treatment plant** is a place where water from nearby rivers and streams is made safe to drink. The water you drink in your home and at school probably comes from a water-treatment plant. At this kind of plant, water is sent through a filter to remove dirt. The water is also treated with certain chemicals. These chemicals kill pathogens, or germs. After being filtered and treated, the water is tested to be sure it is safe to drink. Treated water gets into your home through underground pipes.

Ways You Can Help Reduce Water Pollution

- Do not drink tap water if it is discolored or has a strange odor. Ask your local water company or health department to test the water.

- Use soaps and shampoos whose labels say they are biodegradable. Biodegradable (BY·oh·di·GRAY· duh·buhl) means the soap or shampoo can be broken down into harmless substances.

- Do not pour chemicals on the ground, down the toilet, or down the drain. Do not dump garbage or chemicals into water such as lakes, rivers, or streams.

- Help clean up lakes, rivers, and streams in your community.

How Does Land Pollution Affect My Health?

Land is polluted when people are careless. *Litter* is trash that is thrown on land or in water. Examples of litter are tissues, candy wrappers, and soft drink cans. Litter attracts rats and insects, such as flies, that spread germs to people.

Another way land is polluted is at an open dump. An *open dump* is an area where garbage and wastes are piled. Open dumps attract rats, insects, flies, and mosquitoes. Open dumps stink and are unpleasant to see. Because of health risks, open dumps are being used less often.

Litter and land pollution harm the visual environment. The *visual environment* is everything a person sees regularly. *Visual pollution* is sights that are unattractive. Suppose there is litter in your yard. The litter is unattractive. It pollutes the visual environment. People often throw litter in empty lots. Because no one lives on the land, no one picks up the litter. This creates visual pollution in a neighborhood.

Another cause of land pollution is hazardous waste. *Hazardous waste* is any substance that is harmful to people or animals. Factories create hazardous waste while making products. Chemicals such as paint and motor oil become hazardous waste when people throw them away. Hazardous waste can harm health if it gets into soil. Hazardous waste should be thrown away at special centers.

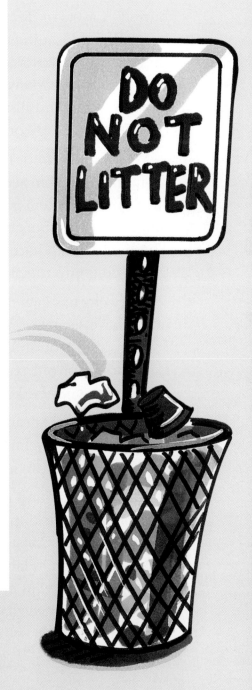

How Can I Help Reduce Land Pollution?

Many communities bury wastes like garbage in landfills. *A landfill* is a place where waste is dumped and buried. Layers of dirt are piled on the waste. This keeps flies, mosquitoes, and rats from coming near the waste. The covered land can then be used for other purposes. Many parks and golf courses have been built on landfills. People often do not know that these parks are on top of a landfill.

Many cities do not have landfills. In these cities, wastes might be burned in an incinerator. An *incinerator* (in·SI·nuh·RAY·ter) is a furnace in which garbage and other wastes are burned. An incinerator has filters. These filters trap harmful products and keep them from going into the air while the wastes are burning.

Every city has laws that help control waste. You might have seen a sign that says DO NOT LITTER. It is illegal for you to litter in your community. You can help keep your community clean by throwing litter into a litter basket.

Another way you can help reduce waste is by recycling, reusing, and precycling. You will learn about these ways to reduce waste in Lesson 39.

Take action if land pollution harms your visual environment. Pick up trash in your yard and neighborhood. Consider forming a group to clean up a park or stream. Plant flowers or vegetables. Suppose there is an empty lot in your neighborhood. Talk to your parents or guardian about planting a community garden with some of your neighbors.

Compost Your Toast

If you have a garden, you might make a compost pile to put nutrients in the soil. *Compost* (KAHM·post) is decayed plant matter that can be used to fertilize soil. Ask your parent or guardian for permission to make a compost pile. Include things like vegetable and fruit peelings and leftover grain products. There are many books on composting. Check one out of the library to learn more.

Pollution Protection

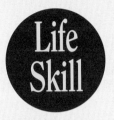

Life Skill

I will help protect my environment.

Materials: Poster paper, markers, pen or pencil

Directions: Follow the directions to find sources of indoor air pollution in your home.

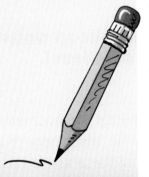

Activity

1. **Draw a map of your home.** Your map should be carefully drawn and as accurate as possible.

2. **On the map, write or draw sources of indoor air pollution that exist in your home.** For example, you might include cigarette smoke, radon, and household chemicals such as cleansers.

3. **Write ways to lower the indoor air pollution in your home on a separate sheet of paper.**

4. **Talk about your map with your parents or guardian.** Make a plan to reduce the indoor air pollution in your home.

Lesson 37

Review

Vocabulary

Write a separate sentence using each of the vocabulary words listed on page 280.

Health Content

Write answers to the following:

1. How does air pollution affect your health? **page 281**

2. What are five ways you can help reduce air pollution? **page 282**

3. How does water pollution affect your health? **page 283**

4. What are four ways you can help reduce water pollution? **page 284**

5. What are six ways you can help reduce land pollution? **page 286**

It's Noisy Out There

Vocabulary

noise pollution: loud or constant noise that causes hearing loss and stress.

decibel: a measure of the loudness of sounds.

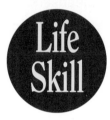

Life Skill

• **I will keep noise at a safe level.**

Think about the sounds you hear every day. You probably hear traffic, machinery, music, and other people. Some of these sounds can harm your hearing. Some of these sounds can cause stress and discomfort. You need to lower your risk of hearing loss and stress from loud sounds.

The Lesson Objectives

• Explain how noise pollution affects your health.

• Discuss ways you can help reduce noise pollution.

How Does Noise Pollution Affect My Health?

Noise pollution is loud or constant noise that causes hearing loss and stress. The louder a sound, the greater the possible harm to a person's body. The lowest sound that can be heard by most people has a decibel of one. A **decibel** (DE·suh·buhl) is a measure of the loudness of sounds. A conversation with another person will measure about 60 decibels. This amount of sound is not harmful. A jet flying overhead might produce a sound of 100 decibels. Sounds above 85 to 90 decibels might cause hearing loss.

You might have hearing loss if you listen to loud noises for a long period of time. The nerve cells in the ears might become damaged.

Loud noises have other effects on your body. Loud noise can cause stress. You might feel nervous. Your heart rate might increase. Suppose you try to study for a test while listening to loud music. You might not be able to keep your mind on your studies.

Hearing many noises at the same time can be confusing, even if each noise is not loud. Again, suppose you try to study for a test. Suppose someone nearby is talking. You might hear a TV from another direction. Someone might be mowing the lawn next door. All these sounds can make it hard to concentrate. You might be distracted by the nearby conversation. You might not be able to study effectively. Plan to study in a quiet place away from distractions. Ask your parents or guardian for permission to study at the library if your home is noisy.

Short-Term Hearing Loss

Suppose you have been near a loud noise for a period of time. You might have ringing in your ears. Your ears might feel full. This means that you have lost your ability to hear some sounds. Usually, this type of hearing loss goes away. But if you continue to be near loud sounds, the hearing loss might become permanent. Follow the directions on page 290 to protect your hearing.

How Can I Help Reduce Noise Pollution?

Think about all the sounds you hear outdoors. You hear jets, buses, and horns from cars. Many outdoor noises are controlled by laws. Many areas have laws that do not allow loud music after a certain hour at night. There are other laws that require that mufflers be used on cars to reduce noise.

Many types of barriers also help lower outdoor noise. Trees and shrubs help lower noise. Fences and walls along expressways help lower traffic noise. Many buildings have soundproof walls. These walls help keep noise outside a building. But not all outdoor noises can be controlled.

Indoor noises are easier to control than noises that are outdoors. You can turn down the volume of your TV, stereo, or radio to reduce indoor noise. Keep the sound low when you listen to music through headphones. Listening to loud music through headphones can cause permanent hearing loss. Wear earplugs when you use power tools or go to concerts. Remember to be considerate of others. Keep all sounds low so you do not bother other people.

There are ways to soundproof a home. Carpet and heavy drapes absorb some sounds. Insulation between walls helps keep sound from entering other rooms.

How do you know if a sound is too loud? A sound is too loud if you have to yell to be heard above it. A sound is too loud if you cannot hear someone who is less than two feet away. A sound is too loud if it makes your ears hurt or ring, or if it makes you feel unsteady or ill. Your radio or stereo is too loud if you are wearing headphones, but other people can hear the music. A sound is too loud if you cannot hear well when the sound stops.

Cover Your Ears!

When you hear a loud sound from which you cannot escape, cover your ears with your hands. Get away from the sound as soon as possible.

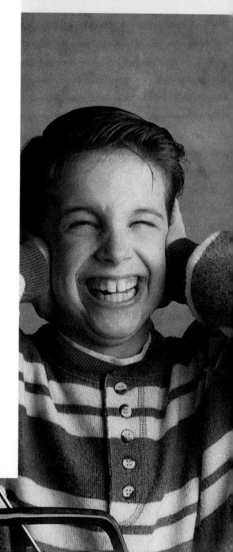

Sounds of Silence

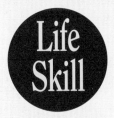

Life Skill I will keep noise at a safe level.

Materials: Paper, pen or pencil

Directions: Follow the directions to become aware of sounds in your environment. Use a separate sheet of paper to write your answers.

Activity

1. **Sit quietly for ten minutes and listen to the sounds around you.** Write down each sound you hear.

2. **Look over the list of sounds you just wrote.** It is likely that some sounds were loud. They might harm your hearing. It is likely that some sounds were not loud, and might have been pleasant to hear.

3. **Make another list next to your first list.** This time, list the sounds in your first list in order from the loudest to the most quiet.

4. **On the back of the sheet of paper, write ways you can lower the three loudest sounds on your list.**

Lesson 38

Review

Vocabulary

Write a separate sentence using each of the vocabulary words listed on page 288.

Health Content

Write answers to the following:

1. How can loud noises harm your hearing? **page 289**

2. What other effects can loud noises have on your body? **page 289**

3. What are two kinds of laws that control outdoor noises? **page 290**

4. What are four ways you can control indoor noise? **page 290**

5. What are six ways you can tell if a sound is too loud? **page 290**

Conserve and Preserve

Vocabulary

conservation: the saving of resources.

energy: the ability to do work.

fossil fuels: coal, oil, and natural gas burned to make energy.

renewable energy: energy whose source can be replaced.

recycling: changing waste products so they can be used again.

reusing: using items again instead of throwing them away and buying new ones.

precycling: taking actions to reduce waste.

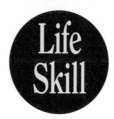

Life Skill

● **I will not waste energy and resources.**

You need to help conserve water and energy. **Conservation** is the saving of resources. When you save resources, you help the environment. You save money. You feel good about yourself because you are being responsible.

The Lesson Objectives

● Discuss ways you can conserve water.

● Discuss ways you can conserve energy.

● Discuss ways you can recycle, reuse, and precycle.

How Can I Conserve Water?

Do you know how much water you use in a day? Think about everything you do with water. You drink it, bathe in it, flush it down your toilet. You wash your clothes and your dishes. Maybe you water your lawn or wash your parents' or guardian's car. Would it surprise you to know that you use about 80 to 100 gallons of water every day?

You might think that there is plenty of water on the earth. In a way, this is true, because water covers about two-thirds of the Earth's surface. But take a look at a globe. Most of the water you see is in oceans. And oceans are salt water, which people cannot drink. People need the fresh water in lakes, rivers, and streams for everyday use. There are many ways you can help conserve water. Here are a few.

Take short showers instead of baths. A quick shower uses much less water than a bath. Time yourself to see how quickly you can get wet, lather up, and rinse. Be careful not to slip and fall!

Run washing machines and dishwashers only for full loads. These appliances use lots of water. Your washing machine might have settings for smaller loads. Use these settings if you have a small load of laundry.

Turn off the faucet while you are washing dishes. Turn it on only to rinse dishes. The same rule applies to toothbrushing. Turn the water on only to rinse your toothbrush and your mouth.

Keep a pitcher of water in the refrigerator if you like to drink cold water. Heat water for tea or hot chocolate on the stove or in the microwave. Letting the faucet run until the water reaches the right temperature wastes water.

Plant trees. Trees store water and release it into the ground.

Did You Know…?

…that 97 percent of the Earth's water is salt water found in oceans and seas?

…that 2 percent of the Earth's water is frozen in ice caps? That is two times the amount of fresh water that is available for people to use!

How Can I Conserve Energy?

Energy is the ability to do work. You use energy every day. The cars and buses you ride in use energy from fossil fuels. **Fossil fuels** are coal, oil, and natural gas burned to make energy. The energy to heat and cool your home and school might come from fossil fuels. Just as you "burn" food to get energy, vehicles and power plants burn fossil fuels to provide energy to you.

Amounts of fossil fuels are limited. Sooner or later, we will run out of them. We will have to find new ways to heat our buildings and fuel our vehicles. People are working on different kinds of renewable energy. **Renewable energy** is energy whose source can be replaced. For example, energy from the sun is renewable, because it arrives every day. We will not run out of energy from the sun. Right now, some people use the sun's energy to heat their homes. As the technology for using the sun's energy becomes better, more people likely will use it. Because fossil fuels do not provide renewable energy, it is important to conserve energy right now. Conserving energy frequently saves money, too. Here are some ways you can conserve energy.

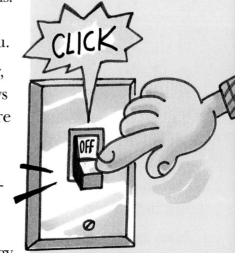

Dress for the weather. Wear a sweater instead of turning up the heat in cold weather. Wear light clothing instead of turning down the air conditioner in hot weather. If practical, use fans instead of air conditioning.

Walk or ride your bike to nearby places instead of asking a parent or guardian to drive you. Get permission from your parents or guardian before you go anywhere by yourself.

Use lights and appliances carefully. Turn off lights when you are the last one to leave a room. Use fluorescent lights or light bulbs with a low wattage except when you read. Fluorescent lights use less energy than standard light bulbs. Use lamps when you read. Turn off your TV, stereo, radio, and curling iron when you are not using them.

Use your own energy. Use manual appliances like can openers and lawn mowers instead of motorized versions.

Follow a...
Health Behavior Contract

Name:_____ **Date:** _____

Life Skill: I will not waste energy and resources.

Effect on My Health: Using less water will help conserve water and keep the water supply safe. Using less water also will help my family save money.

My Plan: I will take short showers instead of baths. I will turn off the faucet while I am washing dishes and brushing my teeth. I will keep a pitcher of water in the refrigerator instead of running the water until it gets cold. I will heat water for tea or hot chocolate on the stove or in the microwave instead of running the water until it gets hot. I will make a mark on my calendar each time I take an action that saves water.

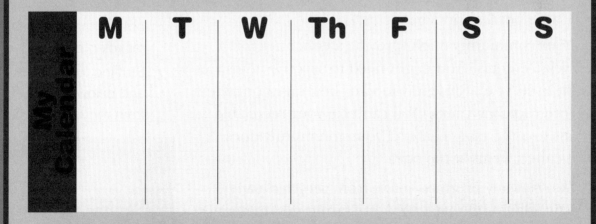

My Calendar	M	T	W	Th	F	S	S

How My Plan Worked: I saved water every day. I feel good about helping the environment.

How Can I Recycle, Reuse, and Precycle?

One way you can keep your community clean is to recycle products that you use. **Recycling** is changing waste products so they can be used again. For example, you might have a soft drink in an aluminum can. Instead of throwing the can away, you can send it to a recycling center. A *recycling center* is a place where waste products are changed so they can be used again. The aluminum can you send to the recycling center could be crushed, and the metal could be used to make more cans. Newspapers might be recycled into products such as boxes and cartons. Many products can be recycled.

Many communities pick up recycled products at the curb. Commonly recycled items include:

• Newspapers, magazines, and office paper
• Cardboard boxes and cartons
• Aluminum cans
• Steel and tin food cans
• Glass bottles and jars
• Plastic bottles and jugs

Your community might provide a container for recyclable items. You might need to sort the items you want to recycle. Rinse any food or beverage containers before recycling them. You can take your recyclable items to a recycling center if your community does not collect items at the curb.

You can buy products made from recycled paper, plastic, glass, and metal. You are saving new material and conserving energy when you buy recycled products. For example, you save trees when you buy products made from recycled paper. Plastic is made from oil, which is not renewable. You save oil when you buy products made from recycled plastic.

Recycled Products You Can Buy

• Notebook paper
• Pencils made from recycled items such as paper, money, clothing, and plastic
• Pens made from recycled paper and plastic
• Bookbags
• Computer disks made from old computer disks
• Mouse pads made from recycled tires
• Garbage cans and bags made from recycled plastic
• Crates and detergent bottles made from recycled plastic
• Stuffing for quilts and pillows made from recycled plastic

You can avoid having to dispose of products if you reuse and precycle. **Reusing** is using items again instead of throwing them away and buying new ones. Think about everything you throw away during a day. Do you throw away glass jars from salsa or peanut butter? You could reuse those jars by storing food in them. You could use them as vases for flowers. You could use them to hold pencils on your desk. You could use them to hold paper clips or other small items.

Do you throw away plastic yogurt cups? You could use them as measuring cups. You could drink out of them. You could put small items in them.

Perhaps you throw away cardboard boxes. You could use those boxes to hold gifts or packages you plan to mail. You could use them to store papers and letters. You could use them to hold things. You could decorate them and store stationary in them. What do you do with old clothing? You could reuse old clothes by giving them to a thrift shop to sell to others. You could use them to make a quilt or a bag.

Precycling

Precycling is taking actions to reduce waste. Precycling involves selecting items with less packaging. Packaging is anything used to wrap or contain a product. For example, buying applesauce in large jars instead of individual-size cups saves resources. Bringing your own cloth bag to the store instead of using the store's plastic bag saves resources. Precycling also involves buying only what you need.

Lesson 39

Review

Vocabulary

Write a separate sentence using each of the vocabulary words listed on page 292.

Health Content

Write answers to the following:

1. What are five ways you can conserve water? **page 293**

2. What are four ways you can conserve energy? **page 294**

3. What are six commonly recycled items? **page 296**

4. What are at least five recycled products you can buy? **page 296**

5. What are at least five ways you can precycle and reuse? **page 297**

Bring Out the Positive

Vocabulary

positive environment: an environment that promotes physical, social, and mental health.

compliment: a positive statement about a person or his or her behavior.

motivate: to encourage someone to do well.

visual environment: everything a person sees regularly.

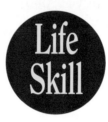
Life Skill

• **I will help keep my environment friendly.**

Is your environment friendly? Do other people encourage you to do your best? Do you help others feel comfortable? A friendly environment improves health. You can help create a friendly environment for yourself and the people around you.

The Lesson Objectives

● Name five characteristics of a positive environment.

● Explain why you should give compliments.

● Tell how you can create a positive environment in your home.

● Explain how poor living conditions affect health.

How Can I Be Positive Around Others?

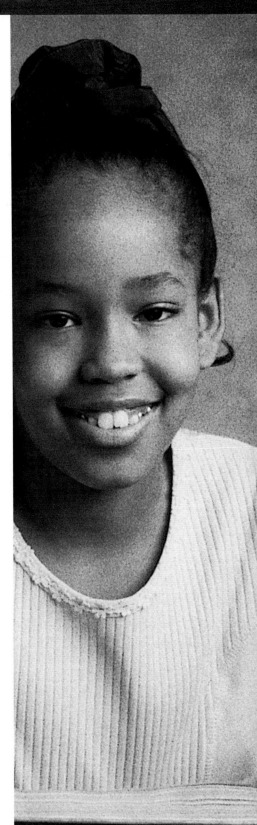

A **positive environment** is an environment that promotes physical, social, and mental health. When you live in a positive environment, you feel safe. You know that other people value your feelings. Other people encourage you to do your best. They do not put you down.

You can help create a positive environment for everyone around you. Give compliments to other people. A **compliment** is a positive statement about a person or his or her behavior. For example, you might tell a classmate that you like his or her outfit. You might congratulate a friend who got an "A" on a test. You might tell your parent or guardian you enjoyed the meal he or she cooked. Compliments make people feel good about themselves. They are pleased that another person has noticed their efforts. Compliments motivate people. To **motivate** is to encourage someone to do well.

Another way to create a positive environment is to avoid giving put-downs. A put-down is a negative statement that makes a person feel bad. Put-downs do not motivate people. Put-downs harm a person's self-confidence. As the old saying goes, "If you don't have anything nice to say, don't say anything."

You can help create a positive environment in your home by helping with chores. Do the dishes without being asked. Make your bed. Clean up your projects in the living room and kitchen. You save work for someone else when you help. One person does not have to do all the work.

A positive visual environment is important, too. The **visual environment** is everything a person sees regularly. Keep your visual environment neat and tidy. Clean up trash in your yard and neighborhood.

How Do Poor Living Conditions Affect Health?

Many people in the world have poor living conditions. Some people do not have enough to eat. Some people live in crowded places. They might be cold in winter and hot in summer. Some people do not feel safe in their environments. There might be people who have weapons. There might be people who abuse others. Some people do not have people who encourage them to do their best.

Poor living conditions can harm health. They can cause stress. They can cause people to get sick more often. They can cause people to choose risk behaviors. People who live in areas where there is violence might be injured or killed. People who are abused might be injured. People who are not encouraged to do their best might give up. They might not work toward their goals.

Take action if you have poor living conditions.
Remind yourself that you deserve a positive environment. Ignore put-downs people give you. Tell yourself you are worthwhile. Set goals and work toward them. For example, you might set a goal of getting at least three "A's" this grading period. Study hard to reach your goal.

Find a mentor. A mentor is a responsible person who helps another person. A mentor can help you work toward your goals. A mentor might be a teacher, a business person, or another trusted adult.

Avoid people who are violent or who use weapons.
Do not choose risk behaviors such as using drugs. Do not use violence or weapons.

Tell a responsible adult immediately if someone abuses you. A responsible adult can help you stop the abuse. Abuse is not the fault of the victim.

Helping Out

There are services to help people who have poor living conditions, but they need volunteers to help them. Ask your parents or guardian about ways you can help people who have poor living conditions. For example, you might collect clothes for people who cannot afford to buy them. You might collect food for people who do not have enough. Your family might volunteer together to serve food at a soup kitchen or shelter.

Warm Fuzzies

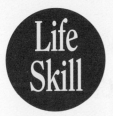

Life Skill

I will help keep my environment friendly.

Materials: Construction paper, markers, scissors

Directions: Follow the directions to promote a positive environment in your home.

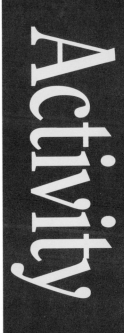

Activity

1. **Make at least ten cards out of construction paper.** Write "Warm Fuzzy" at the top of each card. Leave a blank space on each card in which people can write. Decorate the cards.

2. **Place the cards in a central location in your home.** Explain that family members can write compliments to other family members on the cards. Then they can give the cards to the family members about whom they wrote.

3. **Make more cards if your family uses them up.**

Lesson 40

Review

Vocabulary

Write a separate sentence using each of the vocabulary words listed on page 298.

Health Content

Write answers to the following:

1. What are five characteristics of a positive environment? **page 299**

2. How do compliments promote a positive environment? **page 299**

3. How can you help create a positive environment in your home? **page 299**

4. How do poor living conditions affect health? **page 300**

5. What are four ways you can improve poor living conditions? **page 300**

Unit 9 Review

Health Content

Review your answers for each Lesson Review in this unit. Write answers to the following questions.

1. How can you help reduce water pollution? **Lesson 37 page 284**

2. How does land pollution affect your health? **Lesson 37 page 285**

3. What are five ways loud noises can affect your health? **Lesson 38 page 289**

4. What should you do if you hear a loud sound you cannot escape from? **Lesson 38 page 290**

5. What are two ways you can soundproof your home? **Lesson 38 page 290**

6. How do people use energy from fossil fuels? **Lesson 39 page 294**

7. What is one kind of renewable energy? **Lesson 39 page 294**

8. How should you prepare items for recycling? **Lesson 39 page 296**

9. What are four ways you can help create a positive environment? **Lesson 40 page 299**

10. What are seven ways poor living conditions can harm health? **Lesson 40 page 300**

Guidelines for Making Responsible Decisions™

You decide to wash the dishes. You let the water run while you wash. "It's too much trouble to turn it on and off," you say. Use a separate sheet of paper. Answer "yes" or "no" to each of the following questions. Explain your answer.

1. Is it healthful for you to let the water run while you wash dishes?

2. Is it safe for you to let the water run while you wash dishes?

3. Do you follow rules and laws if you let the water run while you wash dishes?

4. Do you show respect for yourself and others if you let the water run while you wash dishes?

5. Do you follow your family's guidelines if you let the water run while you wash dishes?

6. Do you show good character if you let the water run while you wash dishes?

What is the responsible decision to make?

Multicultural Health

Find a book about living conditions in another country. Read the book. Write a one-page paper about the living conditions in that country.

Vocabulary

Number a sheet of paper from 1–10. Read each definition. Next to each number on your sheet of paper, write the vocabulary word that matches the definition.

pollution	fossil fuels
acid rain	reusing
environment	energy
decibel	compliment
conservation	motivate

1. A positive statement about a person or his or her behavior. **Lesson 40**
2. Using items again instead of throwing them away and buying new ones. **Lesson 39**
3. The presence of substances in the environment that can harm your health. **Lesson 37**
4. The ability to do work. **Lesson 39**
5. A measure of the loudness of sounds. **Lesson 38**
6. To encourage someone to do well. **Lesson 40**
7. The saving of resources. **Lesson 39**
8. Everything that is around you. **Lesson 37**
9. Coal, oil, and natural gas burned to make energy. **Lesson 39**
10. Rainfall that includes pollutants. **Lesson 37**

Health Literacy

Effective Communication

Make a poster that shows ways to conserve water. Hang your poster in your home.

Self-Directed Learning

Find out whether your community has a recycling program. Learn what items the program accepts and how to prepare items for recycling.

Critical Thinking

Why is it important to create a positive environment?

Responsible Citizenship

Form a group to clean up trash in your neighborhood. Get permission from your parents or guardian first.

Family Involvement

Ask your parents about installing special water- and energy-saving devices in your home.

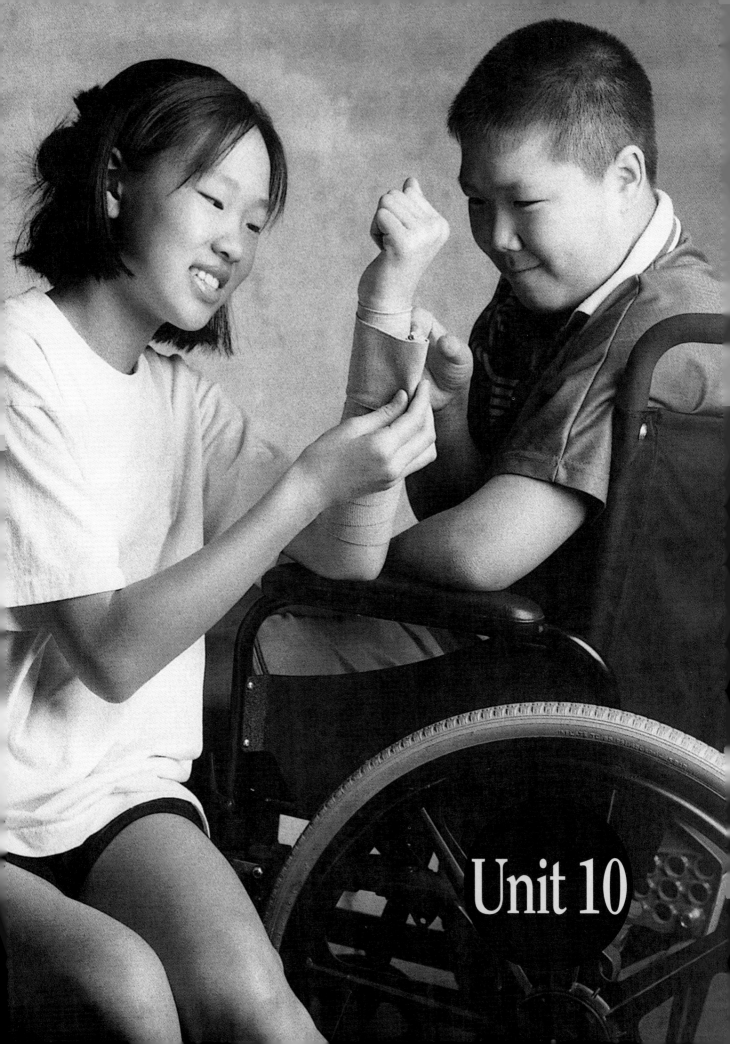

Unit 10

Injury Prevention and Safety

Safety Rules!

Vocabulary

safety rules: guidelines to help prevent injury.

accident: an unexpected event that can result in injury.

smoke detector: a device that sends a signal when smoke is present.

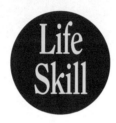

Life Skill

● **I will follow safety rules for my home and school.**

You learn many different facts in school. These facts prepare you for daily living. This lesson contains facts about safety. These facts will help you protect yourself and others from injury. You will learn how you can prevent accidents.

The Lesson Objectives

● Explain why you should follow safety guidelines.

● List safety rules for home, school, and play.

● List safety rules to prevent a fire.

● List safety rules if there is a fire.

Why Should I Follow Safety Rules?

Safety rules are guidelines to help prevent injury. Safety rules are like warning signs. Some warning signs might say, "Walk," "Go," "Do Not Run," "Stop," or "Do Not Enter." These signs are important. They tell you what you should and should not do. These signs help keep you safe from injury. Safety rules work the same way. There are two reasons to follow safety rules.

Follow safety rules to help lower your risk of accidents. An **accident** is an unexpected event that can result in injury. The leading cause of injury to people of all ages is accidents. Most accidents can be prevented. Suppose you are riding your bike in an unsafe way. You do not hold on to the handlebars. You might fall off and get injured. If you had followed safety rules, you might have prevented this accident.

Follow safety rules to help keep others safe. Suppose you leave your skateboard on the sidewalk. Someone could come along and trip over it. That person might fall and become injured. This accident would have been prevented if you had followed safety rules.

You might be tempted to break a safety rule now and then. Suppose you are at a crosswalk. You are in a hurry. The light turns yellow. You run across the street, hoping to beat the light. You might get hit by a car. Being in a hurry is not a good reason to break a safety rule. Suppose a friend dares you to go between two parked cars. This also breaks a safety rule. You might get hit by a car. Taking a dare is not a good reason to break a safety rule. There are no good reasons to break safety rules.

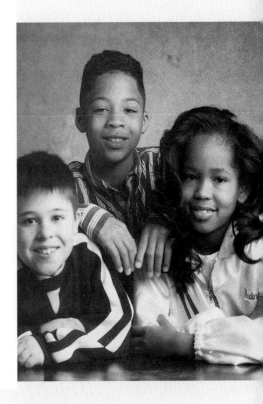

What Are Safety Rules for Home, School, and Play?

Close your eyes and think back to a time when you had an accident. Perhaps you got burned taking food out of the microwave oven. Perhaps you tripped over a book someone in your classroom left on the floor. Perhaps you were building something and hit your thumb with a hammer. You think of your home and school as safe places. Usually they are safe. But accidents happen. You can prevent most accidents. You can follow safety rules for home, school, and play.

Safety Rules for Home

- Keep pathways and stairways clear of toys and books.
- Turn pan handles toward the center of the stove when cooking.
- Use pot holders when removing hot pots, pans, and containers from the stove, oven, or microwave.
- Do not play with matches.
- Do not use electrical items with worn or frayed cords.
- Do not use electrical items when you are wet.
- Do not use power tools unless your parent or guardian is present.
- Follow directions for the safe use of appliances.

Safety Rules for School

- Do not run in hallways.
- Do not push anyone, especially a person who is drinking from a water fountain.
- Keep halls and classroom aisles clear.
- Tell a teacher about wet floors.

Safety Rules for Play

- Use safe and unbroken equipment for play.
- Follow safety rules for all sports and games.
- Always play with a friend when you play outside.
- Tell a parent or guardian where you will be playing.
- Do not play near a construction site.
- Do not play near broken glass.
- Do not play with others who do not follow safety rules.

Follow a...
Health Behavior Contract

Copy the health behavior contract on a separate sheet of paper.

DO NOT WRITE IN THIS BOOK.

Name: ____________________ **Date:** ____________

Life Skill: I will follow safety rules for my home and school.

Effect on My Health: Safety rules are guidelines to help prevent injury. If I follow them, I can prevent accidents. Accidents are the number one cause of injury. I will not be injured. Other people will not be injured. Then I will not miss school. I will not miss out on fun times. I will not feel bad because I broke a rule and someone got hurt.

My Plan: I will use the chart below. I will list five rules to keep me safe at school. Each day of this week (Monday to Friday) I will place a check when I follow a rule.

My Calendar

Safety Rules	M	T	W	Th	F
1.					
2.					
3.					
4.					
5.					

How My Plan Worked: I will use the other side of the health behavior contract. I will write a paragraph about safety rules. I will tell two reasons I should follow safety rules. I will tell which safety rules I think are most important. I will give examples of injuries that can happen if I do not follow safety rules.

What Are Safety Rules for Fires?

Home fires are a major cause of injury. There are many causes. Some fires are caused when a person does not watch food that is cooking. Fires can start when oil or grease becomes very hot or when food spills onto a burner. Some fires are caused by overloaded electrical circuits. Electrical items with damaged cords can cause fires. Some home fires are caused when a person leaves a cigarette burning. The cigarette touches cloth or carpet and starts a fire.

You can follow safety rules to prevent fires.

- Never play with matches.
- Do not run electrical cords under rugs.
- Do not overload electrical outlets.
- Do not leave the room with food cooking on the stove.
- Turn off appliances when you are not using them.
- Have a no smoking policy.
- Have a fire extinguisher in the kitchen.
- Be sure your home has smoke detectors.

A **smoke detector** is a device that sends a signal when smoke is present. The signal warns people to leave a building quickly. Your home should have at least one smoke detector for each level. Check the batteries once a month. Replace dead batteries right away.

How to Call the Fire Department

1. Call 9-1-1.
2. Give your name.
3. Tell the operator there is a fire and that you need help.
4. Tell where the fire is located. Tell the address and nearest cross street.
5. Give the telephone number of the phone you are using.
6. Tell the operator what you know about the fire. Tell if anyone is in danger.
7. Listen carefully to what you are told to do.
8. Do not hang up the phone until the other person has done so.
9. Keep the telephone line clear after the call is complete.

You can follow safety rules if there is a fire. Make a fire escape plan with your parents. Have a plan before a fire starts. Then your family will know what to do if a fire starts. Your plan should show how each person can escape from any room in case of fire. Your plan should show how to safely get out of the house when there is a fire. Your plan should show a meeting place outside your home. All family members should go to that place if a fire starts. Then each member will know whether everyone is safe. Make several copies of your fire escape plan. Post the copies where you can find them easily. Practice your fire escape plan twice a year.

What if a fire starts in your home? Get out right away. Do not stop to get any belongings. Crawl on your hands and knees if there is smoke. Stay below the level of smoke so you do not breathe it. If you are in a room with the door closed, feel the door. If it is hot, do not try to leave. If you are trapped in a room, place blankets or clothes along the edges of the door to keep smoke out. Open a window and yell for help. Wait for firefighters to help you.

Safety Rules for Fires

1. Crawl on your hands and knees.
2. Get out fast!
3. Go to the outdoor meeting place.
4. If a door is hot:
   - do not open the door;
   - place blankets or clothes along the edges of the door;
   - open a window and yell for help.

Lesson 41

Review

Vocabulary

Write a separate sentence using each of the vocabulary words listed on page 306.

Health Content

Write answers to the following:

1. What are two reasons you should follow safety rules? **page 307**
2. What are eight safety rules to follow when you are at home? **page 308**
3. What are four safety rules to follow when you are at school? **page 308**
4. What should you include in a fire escape plan? **page 311**
5. What should you do if a fire starts in your home? **page 311**

Safety Score for the Outdoors

Vocabulary

pedestrian: a person who walks on the sidewalk or in the street.

safety belt: the lap belt and the shoulder belt.

flood: the overflowing of a body of water onto dry land.

hurricane: a tropical storm with heavy rains and winds over 74 miles per hour.

tornado: a violent, spinning windstorm that has a funnel-shaped cloud.

earthquake: a violent shaking of Earth's surface.

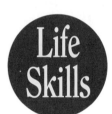
Life Skills

- **I will follow safety rules for biking, walking, and swimming.**
- **I will follow safety rules for riding in a car.**
- **I will follow safety rules for weather conditions.**

When you go to a ball game, do you pay attention to what is going on? Do you know which side is winning? If you do, then you know the score. You also need to pay attention to hazards when you are outdoors. You need to know the score about safety rules when you are outdoors.

The Lesson Objectives

- List safety rules for walking.
- List safety rules for riding a bike.
- List safety rules for swimming.
- List safety rules for riding in a car or bus.
- List safety rules to follow during weather conditions.

What Are Safety Rules for Walking?

A **pedestrian** (puh·DES·tree·uhn) is a person who walks on the sidewalk or in the street. A pedestrian can keep safe by following safety rules. These rules protect people from injuries caused by cars.

Suppose you have to cross a street and a crosswalk is available. Always use the crosswalk. Wait until the traffic signal turns green or the walk sign flashes. Do not cross a street when the traffic light is changing. Some cars try to beat the light and might hit you. If there is no traffic signal, look carefully for traffic. Look left, right, then left again. If no cars are near, you may cross.

Suppose you have to cross a street and there is no crosswalk. If cars are parked nearby, walk to the outer edge of the parked cars. Look left, right, and left again. Cross only if no traffic is coming. Do not dash out and try to beat drivers. Do not enter the street between parked cars.

Suppose you want to walk down a street and there is no sidewalk. Walk near the edge of the street facing traffic. This lets you see cars moving toward you. When possible, walk with a friend or responsible adult. Wear light-colored clothing at dusk and at night.

There is another important safety rule to follow when you are a pedestrian. Never hitchhike! Suppose you and a friend are at the school gym. You are waiting for a parent or guardian to pick you up. Your parent or guardian is late. Do not accept a ride from a person you do not know. Do not start walking in the direction of your home and accept a ride from a stranger. Wait for your parents or guardian. Stay with a responsible adult until your parent or guardian arrives.

Safety Rules for Walking

- Use sidewalks and crosswalks.
- Do not enter the street between parked cars.
- Walk on the side of the road against traffic.
- Walk with a friend or responsible adult.
- Wear light-colored clothing at dusk and at night.
- Do not hitchhike.

What Are Safety Rules for Riding a Bike?

Your bike is like a car if you ride in the street or road. You must follow the same rules as does the driver of a car. This means you must face the same direction as cars. You must ride at a speed that is safe according to the traffic, road conditions, and weather.

People who drive cars must follow many traffic signs. A bike rider also must follow these signs. Know what these signs mean. Use signals to tell drivers of cars when you will stop and what direction you will go.

People who drive cars must watch out for other drivers. You must watch out for drivers, too. Watch for someone opening a car door. Watch for cars and trucks backing out of driveways.

People who drive cars must follow other safety rules. They must keep their cars in good working order. They must wear safety belts. Keep your bike in good working order, too. Wear a safety helmet to protect your head from injury if you fall. Do not ride double. It is hard to control a bike when two people are riding.

Safety Rules for Riding a Bike

- Wear a safety helmet.
- Ride on the same side of the road as do cars.
- Follow traffic signs.
- Place reflector tape on your bike.
- Watch for someone opening a car door.
- Watch for cars and trucks backing out from driveways.
- Keep your bike in good working order.
- Do not ride double.

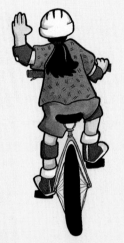
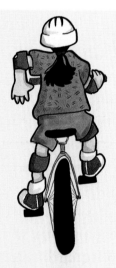

Left turn signal   Right turn signal   Stop

Give correct signals when you are stopping or turning.

What Are Safety Rules for Swimming?

You can have fun in the water when you swim or go boating. However, the water can be dangerous if you do not follow safety rules.

Be safe around water by learning how to swim. Many places hold swimming classes. Always follow safety rules around water. Never swim by yourself. Swim only when a lifeguard is on duty. Do not swim when you are tired. Swim only in good weather. If a storm is coming, get out of the water. Lightning travels through the water. The electricity can harm or kill you if you are in the water.

Diving accidents are a major cause of injury. Dive only where permitted. Never dive into water when you do not know how deep it is. Wait your turn before going off a diving board. Do not horse around a diving board. Do not push people off a diving board.

Swim only in areas where it is safe to swim. Do not swim into an area that is posted NO SWIMMING. Some areas that are posted might have undercurrents. An *undercurrent* is a strong current under the surface of the water. You can get pulled under the water by undercurrents. Do not swim far out when you are in the ocean. Undercurrents can pull you under and away from shore.

Follow safety rules on a boat. Always wear a personal flotation device when you get in a boat. A *personal flotation device (PFD)* is a device that helps you stay afloat. One PFD is a life vest. If you fall in the water, a PFD will help you stay afloat. If your boat tips over, stay near the boat and hold onto it. Yell for help.

Safety Rules for Swimming

- Learn how to swim.
- Always swim with a buddy.
- Swim only when a lifeguard is on duty.
- Do not swim when you are tired.
- Swim only in good weather.
- Dive only where permitted.
- Swim only where swimming is permitted.
- Do not swim far out when you are in the ocean.
- Do not horse around when near water.
- Follow safety rules on a boat.

What Are Safety Rules for Riding in a Car or Bus?

You should follow safety rules when you are a passenger in a car or other motor vehicle. Following these rules will reduce your risk of injury.

Always wear a safety belt even when you are riding a short distance. A **safety belt** is the lap belt and the shoulder belt. Use the safety belt correctly. Make sure it fits snugly. Do not place the shoulder strap behind you. Ride in the back seat. You can be injured by an airbag on the passenger side of the front seat. Lock your door. If you are in an accident, a locked door will be more likely to stay closed than will an unlocked door. Get out on the curb side of a car. You will not get hit by an oncoming car or bike.

Ride only when a car is being driven by a responsible adult. Many car accidents happen when the driver has been drinking alcohol. Do not ride with someone who has been drinking alcohol. Car accidents also can be caused by drivers who speed or race with other drivers. Do not ride with someone who speeds or races with other drivers. Some drivers get so angry with other drivers that they make mistakes when they drive. Do not ride with someone who often gets mad with other drivers.

On a bus, follow rules to help keep you safe. Sit still while the bus is moving. If you stand or move around a lot, you might fall if the bus stops quickly. Do not trip people as they board the bus. Do not yell, scream, throw objects, or get into fights. This might take the driver's attention off the road. Bus drivers must keep their eyes on the road. They must drive the bus safely to keep the students safe.

Safety Rules for Riding in a Car

- Always wear a safety belt.
- Always lock your door.
- Get out on the curb side of a car.
- Ride only with a responsible driver.
- Ride in the back seat to avoid possible air bag injury.

Safety Rules for Riding in a Bus

- Sit still while the bus is moving.
- Do not throw objects.
- Do not make loud noises or yell.
- Do not get into fights.
- Do not trip people who are walking in the aisle.

What Are Safety Rules for Weather Conditions?

You turn on your radio or TV. You hear a weather report about weather conditions where you live. You hear about weather conditions where you do not live. You need to learn safety rules for all types of weather conditions.

Flood

The rain is coming down hard and fast. You hear a warning that rivers might overflow. The announcer forecasts flash floods. A **flood** is the overflowing of a body of water onto dry land. A flood can be very dangerous. Cars and houses can be swept away before people have a chance to get out. You might think it is fun to wade or try to swim in flood water. But people have been swept away trying to swim or drive in flood water. You can follow safety rules during a flood.

- **Leave your home if told to do so.**
- **Do not wade or swim in flood water.**
- **Do not ride in a car or other motor vehicle through flood water.**
- **Turn off all electrical circuits and gas lines if there is a flood.**

Hurricane

Hurricanes are the most powerful storms of all. A **hurricane** is a tropical storm with heavy rains and winds over 74 miles per hour. Hurricanes cause enormous damage. They destroy homes and other buildings, sink ships, and kill people and animals. Many have speeds of over 125 miles per hour and last for days. You can follow safety rules during a hurricane.

- **Follow the warnings by the National Hurricane Service.**
- **Leave the area if you are told to do so.**
- **Call the local chapter of the American Red Cross to find out the location of hurricane shelters.**

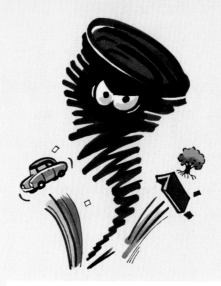

Tornado

Tornadoes are smaller than hurricanes. But their winds are even more powerful. A **tornado** is a violent, spinning windstorm that has a funnel-shaped cloud. A tornado that is no wider than a house can pick up cows and cars. You can stay safe during a tornado.

- **Go to the basement or an underground shelter.**
- **Stay in the center of the ground floor or in a closet if there is no basement.**
- **Stay away from windows.**
- **Get under heavy furniture.**
- **Lie in a low area, such as a ditch, if you are outside.**

El Niño

El Niño is a name for changes in the weather and changes in ocean temperatures around the world. The name "El Niño" means "little boy" in Spanish. El Niño appears every few years and causes good weather and bad weather. It makes winter weather warmer in some places. It also causes many bad weather conditions, such as floods, tornadoes, and hurricanes.

Earthquake

What do you think of when you hear the word "earthquake"? The earth splitting? Bridges crumbling? Dishes breaking? An earthquake can cause all of these. An **earthquake** is a violent shaking of Earth's surface. You can stay safe during an earthquake.

- **Get under a table or desk if you are inside a building.**
- **Stay away from objects that can break or fall.**
- **Stay away from windows and other glass.**
- **Stay away from power lines.**
- **Get out of a car right away.**
- **Get off a bridge right away.**

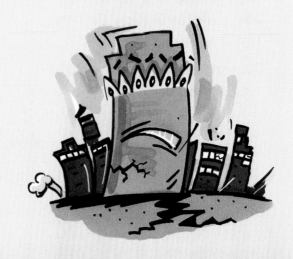

Weather Warning

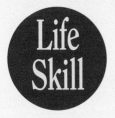

Life Skill

I will follow safety rules for weather conditions.

Materials: Construction paper, markers, scissors

Directions: Learn safety rules in weather conditions.

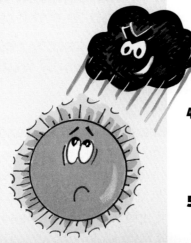

1. **All students will stand by their desks.** Your teacher will choose a student to be a weather announcer. Your teacher will label each of four walls with each weather condition in this lesson.

2. **The weather announcer will call out the name of a weather condition and call on a student.**

3. **The student who is called on must say one safety rule to follow during that weather condition**. The student says the safety rule out loud. The student goes to the wall posted with that weather condition.

4. **When all students have been called on, the students at each wall must create a skit about their weather condition.**

5. **The students must present their skits to the class.**

Lesson 42

Review

Vocabulary

Write a separate sentence using each of the vocabulary words listed on page 312.

Health Content

Write answers to the following:

1. What are safety rules for walking? **page 313**
2. What are safety rules for riding a bike? **page 314**
3. What are safety rules for swimming? **page 315**
4. What are safety rules for riding in a car or bus? **page 316**
5. What are safety rules to follow during weather conditions? **pages 317–318**

Violence-Free

Vocabulary

violence: an act that harms oneself, others, or property.

bullying: hurting or scaring someone younger or smaller.

discrimination: treating some people in a different way than you treat others.

fighting: taking part in a physical struggle.

justice: fairness for all people.

conflict resolution skills: steps you can take to settle disagreements in a responsible way.

victim of violence: a person who is harmed by violence.

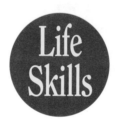

Life Skills

- **I will protect myself from people who might harm me.**
- **I will follow safety rules to protect myself from violence.**

You are growing up in a time when you can find violence almost any place you look. This does not mean violence is okay. Violence is wrong. You need to recognize violence. You need to be able to tell the difference between right and wrong. You need to learn ways to protect yourself from violence.

The Lesson Objectives

- List ways you can recognize violence.
- Explain why you should avoid violence in the media.
- Discuss why you need to follow laws.
- List ways you can express your anger without violence.
- List ways you can stay away from fights.
- Explain how you can get help if you are a victim of violence.

How Can I Recognize Violence?

At recess a girl called another girl a dirty name. In gym class a boy threw a basketball at another boy a little too hard to be an accident. At lunch a bully swiped your chocolate milk. All of these situations involved violence. **Violence** is an act that harms oneself, others, or property. It is wrong to harm yourself or others. It is wrong to damage or destroy property. It is wrong for others to harm you.

Here are some types of violence you need to recognize:

- **Bullying** is hurting or scaring someone younger or smaller. Most people your age have been bullied. A bully makes you get up if he or she wants your seat on the bus. A bully breaks in line at the water fountain. Bullies get away with these actions because they say they will hurt you if you tell or complain. Bullying is violence and it is wrong.

- **Discrimination** is treating some people in a different way than you treat others. Maybe you have called someone who is different an ugly name. Maybe you have told a joke about people of a different race. This is violence. It is wrong. These actions make people angry. They might try to get even. This can lead to violence. Treat all people with respect. When you respect others, you are more likely to get treated the same way. You are less likely to become involved in violence.

- **Fighting** is taking part in a physical struggle. Fighting is dangerous because you might be hurt. Fighting is wrong. There are other ways to work out disagreements.

Stay Safe from Strangers

When you are home:

- Keep windows and doors locked.
- Do not tell anyone that your parents or guardians are not home.
- Do not tell your name or address over the telephone to someone you do not know.

When you are not home:

- Do not talk to strangers who come up to you.
- Yell for help if someone bothers you.
- Run if you think someone is following you.

Why Should I Avoid Violence in the Media?

Turn on your television. You can find programs and news stories that contain violence. Turn on your radio. You can find songs that contain words about violence. Open a newspaper. You can find stories about murders, robberies, or carjackings.

It is dangerous for you to constantly see, hear, and read about violence. You might start thinking violence is okay. You might begin to believe that this is the way everyone acts. Even worse, you might begin to believe it is okay for YOU to act this way.

Let's look at some examples. Michael plays a lot of computer games. His favorite one has a character who goes from place to place shooting and killing people. Michael thinks this character is cool. Michael begins to think shooting is okay. He wants to get a handgun.

Cherise watches lots of movies on videotapes. The women in some movies are treated in wrong ways by men. Cherise begins to think all men treat women in these ways. She gets confused. Now she does not expect boys her age to respect her.

Jacob listens to compact disks with songs about violence. According to Jacob, "My favorite group really rocks. If they say it's okay to beat somebody up, then it must be cool." Jacob wants to be like the members of his favorite group. Jacob starts getting into fights and is suspended from school.

Young people your age who watch or listen to media violence get wrong messages. They might believe wrong messages. Do not let this happen to you. Violence is NOT okay. You can control your actions. You can respect others. You do not have to copy a rock star or movie character whose actions are violent.

Avoid Violence in Media

Here are some ways you can avoid violence in the media.

- Pay attention to ratings of TV programs and movies.
- Do not watch programs with violence.
- Do not listen to songs that tell you violence is okay.

Why Do I Need to Follow Laws?

A *law* is a rule that represents the beliefs of most people in a community, state, or nation. Laws provide order. They help people live together in safe ways. When you follow laws, you and others are safe. Laws provide justice. **Justice** is fairness for all people. When you follow laws, you treat others fairly. Other people who follow laws treat you fairly.

Consider some laws you must follow. One law is about belongings. It is fair for you not to take someone's belongings. It is fair that no one takes yours. You must follow this law to be fair. You should not go into a grocery store and take a candy bar. It is not even OK to take one piece of gum. If you do, you are not fair to the owner of the store. You are stealing.

Suppose you really want a T-shirt at a store. You have your bookbag with you. You think you could slip it into the bookbag without getting caught. This also is stealing. Never break a law because you think you can get away with it.

Suppose you are playing baseball. You bat a ball and it breaks a window. What do you do? Should you run away quickly and pretend it did not

happen? You have damaged someone else's belongings. The laws says you cannot damage someone's property. You must tell the person.

Suppose you see a sign near a creek that says NO TRESPASSING. You want to wade in the creek. Should you sneak on the property? NO, it is against the law. This sign is posted to protect you from harm. It is posted to protect someone's property. You must stay off.

There is something to remember about laws. If you break the law, it is wrong. It is against the law to steal $500. But it also is against the law to steal 25 cents. Set high standards for yourself. Do not try to get away with anything wrong. You need to follow laws.

Laws:

- provide order in your community;
- protect your belongings and those of others;
- provide fairness for all people;
- protect you and others from harm.

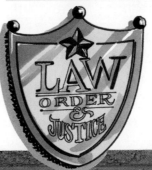

How Can I Express Anger Without Violence?

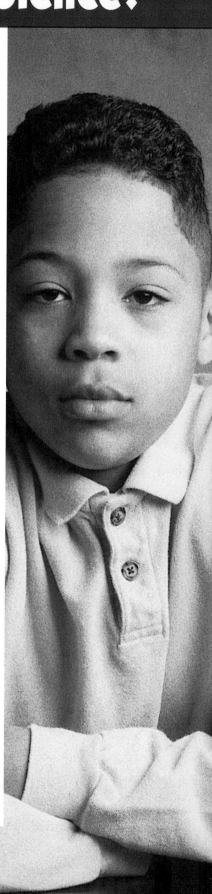

Suppose a friend hides your bookbag at the end of the school day. You almost miss the bus before you find it. You feel angry at your friend. Your friend says you should not feel angry because he or she was only teasing. Should you feel angry?

Anger is the feeling of being irritated or annoyed. You have a right to feel angry. It is OK to feel angry. It is not OK to harm yourself or others when you feel angry. A person who is angry should not hit another person. A person who is angry should not say something mean. A person who is angry should not destroy property.

Express your anger without violence. Here are three ways you can express your anger.

Use I-messages to tell someone what you are feeling.
You might say, "I couldn't find my bookbag. I almost missed the bus and I feel angry." This gives your friend a chance to say he or she is sorry. But what if you say, "You dirtbag! Just wait 'til tomorrow and see what I do to you!" The trouble between you and your friend would grow. You might get into a fight.

Let off steam with healthful physical activity.
Run as fast as you can. Hit a softball as hard as you can. Slam dunk a basketball. Scream into a pillow. You will work off the energy you built up feeling angry. Then you will not blow up and do something you regret.

Write about your feelings.
Write a letter to the person with whom you are angry. Put the letter away for a while. Read it later when you have cooled off. Decide whether you really want to send the letter. You might choose to throw it away. But the act of writing down your feelings helped you manage your anger.

How Can I Stay Away from Fights?

During gym class, Tyler yells to Corey, "Hey Shorty! How does it feel to be the shortest kid in the class?" Corey gets angry and is about to throw a punch before the coach stops him. Has something like this happened to you? Do you know how to stay away from fights?

Fighting is never a good way to settle a problem. Fighting is always wrong. Suppose someone calls you a name or pushes you. You might think you are keeping your self-respect if you fight back. The truth is you lose your self-respect. You take wrong actions by trying to hurt someone.

When you fight back, you are letting someone else control you. Sometimes a person will say or do something mean to try to get you to fight. When you lose your temper or fight, the other person has won. The other person has caused you to act the way he or she wanted you to.

You can take actions to stay away from fights.

Express your anger without violence. Use I-messages. Let off steam with healthful physical activities. Write about your feelings.

Do not make others think you want to fight. Do not tease someone. Do not give nasty looks. Do not shove, push, or trip someone.

Say NO if someone asks you to fight. Say NO in a firm voice to fighting. Give reasons for saying NO. Be certain your behavior matches your words. Keep away from situations in which there will be fights.

Find ways to settle disagreements instead of fighting. **Conflict resolution skills** are steps you can take to settle disagreements in a responsible way.

Walk away. Leave right away if it looks like a fight will begin.

Conflict Resolution Skills

- Remain calm.
- Set the tone.
- Discuss what happened.
- Be honest about what you have said or done to cause the disagreement.
- Use I-messages to let out your feelings.
- Listen to the feelings of the other person.
- List and discuss possible solutions.
- Agree on a solution.
- Keep your word and follow the solution.
- Ask a trusted adult for help if you cannot agree on a solution.

What Can I Do If I Am Harmed by Violence?

A **victim of violence** is a person who is harmed by violence. Suppose someone steals something that belongs to you. Suppose a group of people band together and call you names. Suppose you are beaten up. You might become scared you will be hurt again. You might become depressed or have nightmares.

If you are a victim of violence, you need help to recover. You might need treatment for physical injuries. You might need treatment for mental suffering. You might need family and friends to listen. You need to know that others care about you.

You can be helped in several ways if you are a victim of violence.

You can talk about your feelings. You can talk with your family or friends. You can talk with another trusted adult, such as your school counselor. You can join a group of people who have gone through the same thing.

You can get treatment for physical injuries. You can go to a doctor's office or hospital.

You can get treatment for mental suffering. Suppose someone broke into your house and took your belongings. You might be afraid that your house will be broken into again. Treatment can help you stop being afraid.

A victim who does not get help is at risk for more violence. How does this happen? Suppose a person is hurt again and again. The person might start believing he or she deserves to be hurt. He or she might not try to stop the violence. Or the person might start hurting others because he or she is angry. Get the help you need if you become a victim of violence.

Unsafe Touch

Unsafe touch is a touch that is not right. An unsafe touch is a touch you do not like. Suppose someone touches a private body part. You have a right to tell someone not to touch you. If someone gives you an unsafe touch, tell the person to stop. Yell or scream. Run away from the person. Tell a trusted adult what happened.

Use... Guidelines for Making Responsible Decisions™

Two of your class-mates plan to sneak away at recess and let the air out of a teacher's tire. They say the teacher will not catch them. They ask you to join them.

Use a separate sheet of paper. Answer "yes" or "no" to each of the following questions. Explain each answer.

1. Is it healthful to let the air out of the teacher's tire?

2. Is it safe to let the air out of the teacher's tire?

3. Do you follow rules and laws if you let the air out of the teacher's tire?

4. Do you show respect for yourself and others if you let the air out of the teacher's tire?

5. Do you follow your family's guidelines if you let the air out of the teacher's tire?

6. Do you show good character if you let the air out of the teacher's tire?

What is the responsible decision to make?

Lesson 43

Review

Vocabulary

Write a separate sentence using each of the vocabulary words listed on page 320.

Health Content

Write answers to the following:

1. What are three types of violence and an example of each type? **page 321**

2. What are reasons you should avoid violence in the media? **page 322**

3. Why do you need to follow laws? **page 323**

4. What are three ways you can express your anger without violence? **page 324**

5. What are five ways you can stay away from fights? **page 325**

Ganging Up

Vocabulary

gang: a group of people involved in dangerous and illegal actions.

wanna-be: a young person who is not yet a gang member but wants to be one.

weapon: a device used for violence.

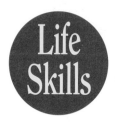

Life Skills

- **I will stay away from gangs.**
- **I will not carry a weapon.**

Kelsey is a fifth grader. She used to take a shortcut home. Then gang members showed up and made her give them money to pass through a certain area. Now Kelsey rides the bus. She does not want anything to do with gangs. A **gang** is a group of people involved in dangerous and illegal actions. You need to stay away from gangs. You need to know how to resist pressure to join a gang.

The Lesson Objectives

- List ways you can recognize gangs.
- Explain why it is risky to belong to a gang.
- Explain how you can be safe from weapons.

How Can I Recognize Gangs?

Suppose a fifth grader in your class wears very baggy pants. Sometimes she wears eyeliner, eyeshadow, and dark lipstick. She puts barrettes in her hair. She draws a special symbol on her notebooks. This student is probably a wanna-be. A **wanna-be** is a young person who is not yet a gang member but wants to be one. It is possible that this fifth grader is already a gang member.

It is important for you to recognize gang members. Then you will know to stay away from them. The following signs might indicate that a person is a gang member.

- The person wears a scarf or item of a certain color all the time.
- The person draws a symbol on objects to show what belongs to the gang.
- The person wears heavy makeup.
- The person hangs out only with other gang members.
- The person uses special hand signs, symbols, and words to communicate with other gang members.
- The person gets a tattoo of the gang's symbol.
- The person gets into trouble, such as by cutting school and getting into fights with teachers.

Why do some young people want to join a gang? There are several reasons. One reason is that a young person might feel lonely. He or she thinks joining a gang will make him or her part of a group. A second reason is that some young people live in an unsafe place. They think other gang members will protect them. A third reason is that some young people want money the easy way. They do not want to have to work for it. They want to steal and sell drugs to get money. A fourth reason is that some young people are bored. They think gang membership is exciting.

Gangs and Drugs

Many gangs are involved in drug trafficking. *Drug trafficking* is the illegal purchase or sale of drugs. Gang members can make a lot of money selling drugs. They use wanna-be's to help them do it. They get wanna-be's to do their dirty work. The wanna-be's might be your age. The wanna-be's look out for police and other adults while the gang members are selling drugs. The wanna-be's try to sell drugs to other students during school hours. Dealing in illegal drugs is very dangerous. Stay away from students who try to sell drugs to you. You do not want anyone to think you want to be a gang member. You could get into trouble with the police. You could get hurt by another gang that thinks you are a gang member.

Why Is It Risky to Belong to a Gang?

There are many reasons it is risky to belong to a gang.

Gang members commit serious crimes. They rob and murder people. They often sell and use illegal drugs. They use illegal weapons and get into fights. They get wanna-be's to commit violent crimes for them. The wanna-be's get into trouble. The gang members do not get caught.

Gang members expect you to behave in wrong and dangerous ways. If you join a gang, you will be involved in illegal drug use. You will be around weapons. You will be pressured to rob, hurt, or even kill other people.

You will be hurt. When you first join a gang, you will have to prove yourself. You might be beaten up by other gang members to see how tough you are. You might have to steal or sell drugs. You might have to hurt other people. Gang members often fight with other gang members. You will be expected to fight, too.

You risk destroying your future. You might be suspended from school or put in jail. You might find it hard to finish school or to get a job. You will have to live with the fact that you have hurt other people.

You will have a hard time leaving the gang. It is almost impossible to leave a gang. You know too much about gang members. The members of your gang might injure or even kill you if you try to leave. They might threaten or hurt your family.

You are not too young to be pressured to join a gang. Prepare now to stay away from gangs.

1. Stay away from gang members.
2. Stay away from places where gang members hang out.
3. Do not wear the same clothes or colors as do gang members.
4. Do not write the symbol of a gang on anything.
5. Do not take part in writing graffiti.
6. Do not use alcohol or other harmful drugs.
7. Do not stay out late at night.
8. Attend school and school activities.
9. Spend time with your family.
10. Say NO and walk away if someone pressures you to join a gang.

Graffiti and Gangs

Graffiti is markings on items that can be seen by others. Gangs communicate their messages through graffiti. They often use signs and symbols. Graffiti might be a warning to other gangs. Graffiti might be a message to other members in the gang. Students who are gang members might write graffiti on school items. Stay away from people who write graffiti. They might be gang members.

Speak Out Against Gangs

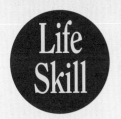

I will stay away from gangs.

Materials: Pencil and two index cards per student

Directions: This activity will help you learn how to stay away from gangs.

I Will Not Join a Gang!

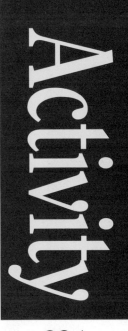

1. **Count off from one to ten.** Match your number to the number of a way you can stay away from gangs above. Copy that way on to one index card.

2. **Write one of the wrong things a gang member might do on the other index card.**

3. **Your teacher will collect and read each card out loud.** When he or she reads a way to stay away from gangs, the class will respond, "STAY AWAY"! When he or she reads a wrong action by a gang member, the class will respond, "I WILL NOT JOIN A GANG"!

How Can I Be Safe from Weapons?

A **weapon** is a device used for violence. You probably think of guns, razor blades, and knives as weapons. Anything can be a weapon if it is used to harm another person. You increase your risk of violence if you carry a weapon. You increase your risk of violence if you do not know how to stay safe from weapons.

Guns are the weapons used most often to harm young people. One reason is they are easy to get. Many young people say they know where to buy a gun. Selling guns to young people under 18 is illegal. However, young people can buy them illegally.

Why do young people buy or carry guns? Some say they are afraid of being attacked. They feel they can defend themselves with a gun. Some say it makes them feel important. Some say they want to protect themselves from people who bully them and from gang members.

It is dangerous for a person to carry a gun or other weapon. If the person gets into a fight, he or she might use the gun or other weapon and injure or kill the other person. If the person had not had the weapon, he or she would have settled the disagreement differently.

It is dangerous for you to be around a weapon. Someone might become angry at you and harm you on purpose. Or someone might harm you accidentally. The person might think a gun was not loaded and aim it at you. Suppose the gun was loaded and the person pulled the trigger. You would be injured or killed.

Never pretend to have a weapon. For example, you might put a hand in your pocket and point a finger. Someone else might think your weapon is real and hurt you in self-defense.

You can be safe from weapons.

1. Do not hang out with people who carry weapons.
2. Do not pick up a weapon. Never think a gun is unloaded.
3. Do not pretend you have a weapon.
4. Do not argue with someone who has a weapon—get away from the person.
5. Do not put yourself in a situation where people will have weapons.
6. Tell an adult if you find a weapon.
7. Do not touch a weapon in your home or someone else's home. The law permits owning handguns or rifles if the owner has a license. Your parents or guardian might have a handgun or rifle. But it is not okay for you to touch it!

Being Responsible Around Weapons

You are at a friend's house. Your friend says he has something special to show you. You go to his parents' bedroom. He opens a drawer. You see a handgun. Your friend says, "Go ahead, pick it up. Pretend you're a detective in a TV show." What is the responsible decision? What should you say to your friend?

Lesson 44

Review

Vocabulary

Write a separate sentence using each of the vocabulary words listed on page 328.

Health Content

Write answers to the following:

1. What are ways you can recognize gangs? **page 329**
2. What are four reasons a young person might join a gang? **page 329**
3. Why is it risky to belong to a gang? **pages 330–331**
4. What are reasons a young person might carry a weapon? **page 332**
5. What are seven ways you can protect yourself from weapons? **page 333**

A Guide to First Aid

Vocabulary

first aid: the temporary care given to a person who has a sudden illness or injury.

emergency: a situation in which help is needed quickly.

unconscious: the condition of not being aware of surroundings.

universal precautions: steps taken to keep from having contact with pathogens in body fluids.

poison: a substance that causes harm if it enters the body.

choking: being unable to breathe.

fracture: a break in a bone.

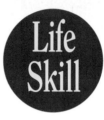

● **I will be skilled in first aid.**

First aid is the temporary care given to a person who has a sudden illness or injury. You should learn first aid for several reasons. You can help others who become ill or injured. You can help yourself if you become ill or injured. You can lower your risk of injury because you will be more careful.

The Lesson Objectives

● Describe when you should call a local emergency number.

● Explain how to make an emergency phone call.

● Explain where you should keep a first aid kit.

● Explain how to use universal precautions when giving first aid.

● List the steps to give first aid for: nosebleeds, scrapes, cuts, punctures, poisoning, choking, fractures, bee stings, bruises, burns and blisters, objects in the eye, skin rashes from plants, and sunburn.

How Can I Be Ready to Give First Aid?

You must be ready to give first aid. You must take four actions if you or someone else is injured.

Action 1

Decide whether to call your local emergency number.

Some injuries are minor. They are not emergencies. You can take care of minor injuries. An **emergency** is a situation in which help is needed quickly. The person who is injured needs to get to an emergency room. You need to know the difference between a minor injury and an emergency. In most places, the local emergency number is 911. You also can call 0 for a telephone operator. The operator can connect you with emergency services in your area. Call 9-1-1 immediately if a person:

- has a hard time breathing or stops breathing;
- has bad chest pain or pressure in the chest;
- has bleeding that will not stop;
- coughs or vomits blood;
- has a broken bone;
- has very bad pain;
- becomes unconscious after an accident or injury.

Unconscious (uhn·KAHN·shuhs) is the condition of not being aware of surroundings. However, the person is not sleeping.

As you read this lesson, you will learn other situations in which you should call 9-1-1.

What to Do for a Badly Injured Person

1. Call 9-1-1.
2. Do not move the person.
3. Cover the person with a blanket.
4. Stay with the person.
5. Keep the person calm.

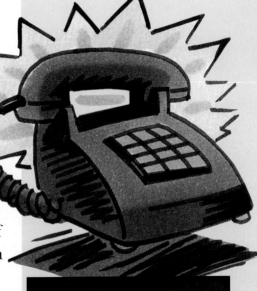

Emergency!
Call 9-1-1 and get medical care immediately.

Action 2
Make an emergency phone call.

Suppose you decide you need to call 9-1-1. Tell the person who is injured that you will get help. Get an adult if one is nearby. If no one is nearby, you will need to make an emergency phone call.

1. Call 9-1-1.
2. Give your name.
3. Tell the operator a person has been injured and needs help.
4. Give the address where help is needed. If you do not know the address, describe the location.
5. Give the telephone number of the phone you are using.
6. Tell what happened and what has already been done.
7. Listen carefully to what you are told to do.
8. Do not hang up until the other person has done so.
9. Return to the injured person. Tell him or her that help is on the way.

Action 3
Find a first aid kit.

You can buy a first aid kit at a drugstore or from the American Red Cross. You should always know where to find a first aid kit. You do not want to waste time looking for one when someone is hurt. Keep a first aid kit in your home and in the family car. Make sure everyone knows where it is. Take a first aid kit with you when you are playing outdoors away from home.

Action 4
Give first aid for injuries and illnesses.

Use universal precautions.

How to Use Universal Precautions

HIV is the pathogen that causes AIDS. HIV is found in blood. Maybe the person who is injured has HIV. Maybe he or she does not. You cannot tell just by looking at the person. Be safe and use universal precautions when giving first aid. **Universal precautions** are steps taken to keep from having contact with pathogens in body fluids.

1. Wear disposable latex or vinyl gloves.
2. Do not wear the same gloves more than once.
3. Wash your hands with soap and water after you take off the gloves.
4. Do not eat or drink anything while giving first aid.
5. Do not touch your mouth, eyes, or nose while giving first aid.

What Is First Aid for Bleeding and Poisoning?

Bleeding

You usually can treat a nosebleed by yourself. The person with the nosebleed should sit forward in a chair. He or she should pinch the nostrils together for five to ten minutes. The person should breathe from the mouth and spit out any blood.

A *scrape* is a wearing away of the outer layer of the skin. Scrapes usually are minor injuries and do not bleed much. Clean the area with soap and water. Place a clean bandage over the scrape. This helps control bleeding and prevent infection.

Another common wound is a cut. You can use first aid skills for a minor cut. Clean the cut with soap and water. Put pressure on the cut with a bandage if the cut bleeds. Cover the cut with a clean bandage.

A *puncture* (PUHNK·cher) is a wound in which something goes deep through the skin and makes a hole. A puncture wound damages tissue deep inside the body. Pins, nails, or an animal bite can cause a puncture wound. Clean the area with soap and water. Tell an adult if you get a puncture wound.

Tetanus (TET·nuhs) is an infection caused by poisons from bacteria that have entered a wound. This disease attacks the nervous system. You should see a doctor if you get a puncture wound. You should go even if you are up-to-date on your tetanus vaccines. You might need a booster vaccine.

Poisoning

A **poison** is a substance that causes harm if it enters the body. You can be poisoned by eating, drinking, breathing, or getting poisons on your skin. If you think someone has been poisoned, call 9-1-1 right away. Try to find out what the poison is. Save the container. Do not make the person vomit unless you are told to do so by a medical professional.

Emergency!
Call 9-1-1 if bleeding does not stop.

Follow Universal Precautions

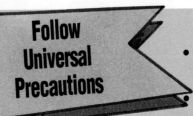

- **Wear Disposable Latex Gloves**
- **Always Use a Face Mask**

What Is First Aid for Choking and Fractures?

Choking

Choking is being unable to breathe. A person can choke when food or a small object gets caught in the windpipe. A person who is choking needs help RIGHT AWAY! The person might put a hand to his or her throat. This is the sign for choking. The person will not be able to talk. Tell the person to cough several times. If the person cannot cough up the object, you will need to give first aid.

If someone is choking, stand behind the person. Place the thumb of your fist above the person's navel. Wrap your other hand around your fist. Press into the abdomen up toward the ribcage with a quick, upward thrust. Repeat until the object comes out.

Fractures

A **fracture** is a break in a bone. Most fractures are caused by falls and accidents. There are many different kinds of fractures. One kind of fracture is a crack in the bone. Another kind of fracture is a complete break of a bone into two pieces.

How does a person know if a bone has been fractured? A person might hear or feel a bone snap. The injured area might be painful and swollen. The area might look purple. Part of a bone might stick out of the skin.

If you think someone has a fracture, do not move the injured body part. You might cause the broken bone to move. The broken bone might harm other body tissues. Place ice over the injured area to reduce swelling. Call 9-1-1. The best way to know if a person has a fracture is to have an X-ray taken. The X-ray will help a doctor know if the bone is broken and where the break is.

Emergency!
Call 9-1-1 and get medical care immediately.

What Is First Aid for Minor Injuries?

Bee Stings

A honeybee will leave its stinger in the skin. The stinger will continue to inject venom for about two or three minutes. Venom is the poison that is injected into a person's body from an insect or animal. Remove the stinger as soon as possible. Flick it out with a nail file or a similar object. Do not pull out the stinger with your finger. You might squeeze more venom out. When the stinger is out, clean the area with soap and water. Place ice over the area to relieve pain and swelling. Tell an adult you have been stung. Call 9-1-1 if a person has trouble breathing, turns blue, or the area around a sting swells. The person might be having an allergic reaction.

Emergency!
Call 9-1-1 if a person cannot breathe, turns blue, or the stung area swells.

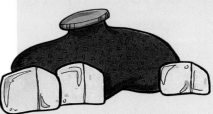

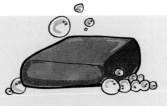

After a bee sting is removed, clean the area with soap and water.

Place an ice pack on a bruise for ten minutes.

Bruises

A *bruise* (BROOZ) is an area under the skin into which blood has leaked. Place a cold cloth or ice pack on the bruise for ten minutes. See a doctor if the bruise does not go away in a week. A black eye is bruised skin around the eye. Place a cold cloth over the area for ten minutes. Do not put a cloth or bag directly on the eye. See a doctor to make sure the eye is not damaged.

See a doctor if a bruise does not go away in a week.

See a doctor if you get a black eye.

Burn

A *burn* is an injury caused by heat, electricity, chemicals, or radiation. You can treat a minor burn. Place a cold cloth over the burn or place the burned area under cold running water for ten minutes. Cover the area with a clean bandage. See a doctor if the burn turns more red, has pus, or swells.

Blister

A *blister* is an area on the skin where fluid has collected. A blister can be caused by a burn or rubbing against the skin. Clean a blister with soap and water. Place a clean bandage on it. Do not break the blister. See a doctor if the area becomes more red, has pus, or swells.

Objects in the Eye

Never rub your eye if anything gets in it. You might harm your eyesight. Tell an adult. The adult should rinse the eye by gently pouring water on the eye. See a doctor if the object does not come out.

Skin Rashes from Plants

Poison ivy, poison oak, and poison sumac can cause skin rashes. The skin might itch, burn, and turn red. The sap from these plants causes an allergic reaction in some people. If you get a rash from a plant, do not scratch or rub the rash. Use an over-the-counter product to relieve the itching.

Sunburn

Stay out of the sun if you become sunburned. Place cloths soaked in cold water on the parts that hurt the most. Do not break blisters. If the blisters break, wash the area with soap and water each day. Cover the area with clean gauze to prevent infection. See a doctor if the burned area becomes more red, has pus, or swells.

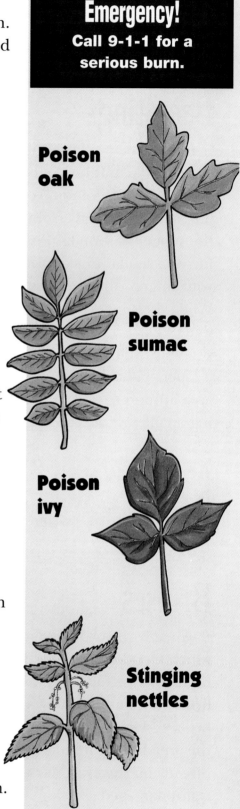

Emergency!
Call 9-1-1 for a serious burn.

Poison oak

Poison sumac

Poison ivy

Stinging nettles

My Quick First Aid Guide

Person Who Is Badly Injured

1. Call 9-1-1.
2. Do not move the person.
3. Cover the person with a blanket.
4. Stay with the person.
5. Keep the person calm.

Nosebleed

1. Sit forward in a chair.
2. Pinch the nostrils together.
3. Breathe through the mouth.
4. Spit out any blood.
5. Call 9-1-1 if bleeding does not stop.

Scrape

1. Clean the area with soap and water.
2. Place a clean bandage over the scrape.

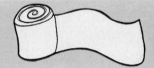

Cut

1. Clean the cut with soap and water.
2. Apply pressure with a clean bandage if the cut is bleeding.
3. Cover the cut with a clean bandage.
4. Call 9-1-1 if bleeding does not stop.

Puncture

1. Clean the area with soap and water.
2. Tell an adult.
3. See a physician.

Poisoning

1. Call 9-1-1.
2. Find out what the poison is.
3. Find out how much poison entered the person.
4. Save the container.
5. Do not make the person vomit unless a medical person tells you to do so.

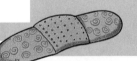
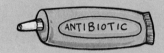

Choking (if someone else is choking)

1. Stand behind the choking person.
2. Make a fist with one hand.
3. Place the thumb of your fist above the person's navel.
4. Wrap your other hand around your fist.
5. Press into the abdomen up toward the ribcage with a quick, upward thrust.
6. Repeat until the object comes out.
7. Call 9-1-1 if the object does not come out.

Choking (if you are choking)

1. Try to get someone's attention.
2. Grab your throat to show you are choking.
3. If you are alone, make a fist with one hand.
4. Grab the fist with your other hand.
5. Press into your abdomen up toward the ribcage with a quick, upward thrust.
6. Repeat until the object comes out.

Fracture

1. Do not move the injured part.
2. Place ice over the injured part.
3. Call 9-1-1.

Bruise

1. Place a cold cloth on the bruise for ten minutes.
2. Do not put a cloth directly on a black eye.

Bee Sting

1. Remove the stinger.
2. Clean the area with soap and water.
3. Put ice over the area.
4. Tell an adult.
5. Call 9-1-1 if the person cannot breathe, turns blue, or the stung area swells.

Skin Rashes from Plants

1. Do not scratch or rub the rash.
2. Use an over-the-counter product to relieve the itching.

Burn

1. Place a cold cloth over the burn or place the burn under cold running water for ten minutes.
2. Cover the area with a clean bandage.
3. Call 9-1-1 for serious burns.
4. See a doctor if a minor burn gets worse.

Blister

1. Clean the area with soap and water.
2. Place a clean bandage over the blister.
3. Do not break a blister.
4. See a doctor if the blister gets worse.

Objects in the Eye

1. Do not rub your eye.
2. Tell an adult.
3. The adult will pour water on the eye.
4. See a doctor if the object does not come out.

Sunburn

1. Stay out of the sun.
2. Place cloths soaked in cool water on burned areas or take a cool shower.
3. Clean the area with soap and water if blisters break.
4. Do not break blisters.
5. Cover the area with clean gauze if blisters break.
6. See a doctor if the burned areas get worse.

Race to the Rescue

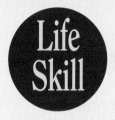

Life Skill

I will be skilled in first aid.

Materials: Paper, markers, scissors, tape

Directions: Help your teammates race to the rescue.

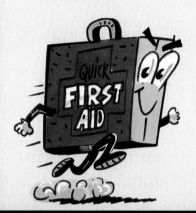

Activity

1. **Your teacher will divide your class into two teams.** He or she will assign each student steps from My Quick First Aid Guide. Each team will write a complete set of first aid steps.

2. **Write each step in big letters.** Cut the steps into strips. Your teacher will collect, mix up, and pass out a complete set of first aid steps to each team.

3. **Your teacher will post the names of injuries for each team.** Students will take turns placing their strips under the correct injuries. Students from both teams will take turns at the same time. The team that completes its Quick First Aid Guide first wins.

Lesson 45

Review

Vocabulary

Write a separate sentence using each of the vocabulary words listed on page 334.

Health Content

Write answers to the following:

1. When should you call your local emergency number? **page 335**

2. What are the steps to make an emergency phone call? **page 336**

3. Where should you keep a first aid kit? **page 336**

4. How can you keep from getting HIV when giving first aid? **page 336**

5. What are the steps to give first aid for: nosebleeds, scrapes, cuts, punctures, poisoning, choking, fractures, bee stings, bruises, burns, blisters, objects in the eye, skin rashes from plants, and sunburn? **pages 337–340**

Unit 10 Review

Health Content

Review your answers for each Lesson Review in this unit. Write answers to the following questions.

1. How can you prevent accidents at home? **Lesson 41 page 308**

2. What should you do if a fire starts in your home? **Lesson 41 page 311**

3. How can you be safe while you are walking? **Lesson 42 page 313**

4. How can you be safe while you are riding a bus? **Lesson 42 page 316**

5. Why should you avoid violence in the media? **Lesson 43 page 322**

6. What actions can you take to stay away from fights? **Lesson 43 page 325**

7. What are signs a person might be a gang member? **Lesson 44 page 329**

8. What are reasons it is risky to join a gang? **Lesson 44 pages 330–331**

9. Where are places you should keep a first aid kit? **Lesson 45 page 336**

10. What are the steps for universal precautions? **Lesson 45 page 336**

Guidelines for Making Responsible Decisions™

A friend's older brother gave your friend a switchblade knife. Your friend wants to show you how to use it. Use a separate sheet of paper. Answer "yes" or "no" to each of the following questions. Explain each answer.

1. Is it healthful for you to handle the knife?

2. Is it safe for you to handle the knife?

3. Do you follow rules and laws if you handle the knife?

4. Do you show respect for yourself and others if you handle the knife?

5. Do you follow your family's guidelines if you handle the knife?

6. Do you show good character if you handle the knife?

What is the responsible decision to make?

Family Involvement

Draw the rooms in your house. Ask your parents or guardian to help you make a fire escape plan for your home.

Vocabulary

Number a sheet of paper from 1–10. Read each definition. Next to each number on your sheet of paper, write the vocabulary word that matches the definition.

accident	fracture
bullying	tornado
gang	unconscious
justice	pedestrian
poison	violence

1. A break in a bone. **Lesson 45**
2. Hurting or scaring someone younger or smaller. **Lesson 43**
3. Fairness for all people. **Lesson 43**
4. A substance that causes harm if it enters the body. **Lesson 45**
5. An unexpected event that can result in injury. **Lesson 41**
6. A group of people involved in dangerous and illegal actions. **Lesson 44**
7. A person who walks on the sidewalk or in the street. **Lesson 42**
8. Harm to oneself, others, or property. **Lesson 43**
9. A violent, spinning windstorm that has a funnel-shaped cloud. **Lesson 42**
10. The condition of not being aware of surroundings. **Lesson 45**

Health Literacy

Effective Communication

 Talk to a coach or physical education teacher at your school. Find out the most common sports injuries and ways to prevent them.

Self-Directed Learning

 Write or call your local American Red Cross chapter. Ask for a pamphlet on swimming safety.

Critical Thinking

 A classmate is thinking about joining a gang. He or she says he or she feels left out and lonely. How can you make this person feel part of a group that is not a gang?

Responsible Citizenship

 Ask permission to visit a classroom of younger students. Show them how to make correct hand signs for bicycle safety.

Multicultural Health

Talk to someone from a country different from yours. Find out what the penalties are for stealing. Compare them to those in your country.

Glossary

Sound	As in	Symbol	Example
ă	cat, tap	a	calculus (KAL·kyuh·luhs)
ā	may, same	ay	atria (AY·tree·uh)
a	wear, dare	ehr	bone marrow (MEHR·oh)
ä	father, top	ah	isotonic (eye·suh·TAH·nik)
ar	car, park	ar	artery (AR·tuh·ree)
ch	chip, touch	ch	choking (CHOH·king)
ĕ	bet, test	e	cerebellum (ser·uh·BEL·uhm)
ē	pea, need	ee	emphysema (em·fuh·SEE·muh)
er	perk, hurt	er	growth spurt (SPERT)
g	go, big	g	ligaments (LIG·uh·muhnts)
ĭ	tip, live	i	cilia (SI·lee·uh)
ī	side, by	y, eye	gingivitis (jihn·juh·VY·tuhs)
j	job, edge	j	school psychologist (SY·KAH·luh·jist)
k	cook, ache	k	quackery (KWA·kuh·ree)
ō	bone, know	oh	alveoli (al·vee·OH·ly)
ô	more, pour	or	hormone (HOR·mohn)
ȯ	saw, all	aw	audiologist (AW·dee·AH·luh·jist)
oi	coin, toy	oy	steroids (STEHR·oydz)
ou	out, now	ow	power (POW·er)
s	see, less	s	cerebrum (suh·REE·bruhm)
sh	she, mission	sh	shadowing (SHA·doh·ing)
ŭ	cup, dug	uh	medulla (muh·DUH·luh)
u	wood, pull	u	bullying (BUL·ee·ing)
ü	rule, union	oo	nutrient (NOO·tree·uhnt)
w	we, away	w	water (WAH·ter)
y	you, yard	yu	stimulants (STIM·yuh·luhnts)
z	zone, raise	z	physician (fuh·ZI·shun)
zh	vision, measure	zh	decision (di·SI·zhuhn)
ə	around, mug	uh	respiratory (RES·puh·ruh·TOR·ee)

A

abstinence (AB·stuh·nuhnts): choosing not to be sexually active.

accident: an unexpected event that can result in injury.

acid rain: rainfall that includes pollutants.

acne: a skin disorder in which pores in the skin are clogged with oil.

acute (uh·KYOOT) **period:** the time during which symptoms of disease are the greatest.

addiction: a strong desire to do something even though it is harmful.

adopt: to take a child of other parents into your family.

advertisement (ad): a paid announcement.

advertising: a form of selling products and services.

aerobic (uhr·OH·bik) **exercise:** exercise that uses a lot of oxygen for a period of time.

age: to grow older.

agility (uh·JI·luh·tee): the ability to move and change directions.

AIDS: a breakdown in the body's ability to fight infection.

Al-Anon: a recovery program for people who are close to someone who has an addiction.

Alateen: a recovery program for teens who are close to someone who has an addiction.

alcohol: a depressant drug found in some beverages.

alcohol-free: to say NO to using alcohol and to going to parties where there is alcohol.

Alcoholics Anonymous (AA): a recovery program for people who have alcoholism.

alcoholism (AL·kuh·HAW·LI·zuhm): a disease in which a person is dependent on alcohol.

allergen: a substance that causes an allergic reaction.

allergist: a doctor who treats people with allergies.

allergy (AL·uhr·jee): the reaction of the body to certain substances.

alveoli (al·vee·OH·ly): small air sacs in the lungs.

amphetamine (am·FE·tuh·MEEN): a stimulant drug used to treat sleep disorders and attention problems.

anabolic steroids: drugs that act like the male hormone testosterone.

anaerobic (an·uhr·OH·bik) **exercise:** exercise that is done for a short time and uses a lot of oxygen.

anger: the feeling of being irritated or annoyed.

angina pectoris (an·JY·nuh PEK·tuhr·uhs): chest pain caused by a lack of oxygen in the heart.

anorexia (a·nuh·REK·see·uh): an eating disorder in which a person starves himself or herself.

antibody: a substance in the blood that helps fight pathogens.

antiperspirant (an·tee·PUHR·spuh·ruhnt): a grooming product used under the arms that reduces the amount of perspiration.

appeal: a statement used to get consumers to buy a product or service.

artery: a blood vessel that carries blood away from the heart.

arthritis (ar·THRY·tis): the painful swelling of joints in the body.

asthma (AZ·muh): a chronic disease in which the small airways get narrow.

atria (AY·tree·uh): the upper parts of the heart.

attitude: your way of thinking and seeing things.

audiologist (AW·dee·AH·luh·jist): a person who tests hearing.

audiometer (AW·dee·AH·muh·ter): a machine used to test hearing.

B

bacteria (bak·TEER·ee·uh): one-celled living things.

balance: the ability to keep from falling.

balanced diet: a daily diet that includes the correct number of servings from the food groups in the Food Guide Pyramid.

barbiturate (bar·BI·chuh·ruht): a drug that relieves anxiety and causes sleepiness.

beta-endorphins (BAY·tuh·en·DOR·fuhns): substances that produce feelings of well-being.

Better Business Bureau (BBB): a group that encourages businesses to treat customers fairly.

binge (BINJ) **eating disorder:** frequently stuffing oneself with food.

blackout: a period about which a person cannot remember what happened.

blister: an area on the skin where fluid has collected.

blood alcohol level (BAL): the amount of alcohol in a person's blood.

blood pressure: the force of blood against the artery walls.

body composition: the amount of fat tissue and lean tissue in your body.

body defenses: ways the body works to protect against pathogens.

body image: the feeling you have about the way your body looks.

body system: a group of organs that work together to carry out certain tasks.

bonding: a process in which two people develop feelings of closeness for one another.

bone marrow (MEHR·oh): the soft tissue in the middle of long bones.

boredom: the state of being restless because you have no interests.

braces: wires used to move the jaws and teeth.

Braille (BRAYL) **system:** a way of touch reading and writing used by a person who is blind.

bronchi (BRAHN·ky): short tubes that carry air from the trachea to both the left and right lung.

bruise (BROOZ): an area under the skin into which blood has leaked.

budget: a plan for spending and saving money.

bulimia (boo·LEE·mee·uh): an eating disorder in which a person stuffs himself or herself and then tries to rid the body of food.

bullying: hurting or scaring someone younger or smaller.

burn: an injury caused by heat, electricity, chemicals, or radiation.

C

caffeine: a stimulant found in chocolate, coffee, tea, some soda pops, and some drugs.

calculus (KAL·kyuh·luhs): hardened plaque.

calorie: a unit of energy produced by foods and used by the body.

cancer: a disease in which cells multiply in ways that are not normal.

capillaries (KA·puh·lehr·eez): small blood vessels that connect arteries to veins.

carbon monoxide (KAR·buhn muh·NAHK·SYD): a poisonous gas that you cannot see or smell.

carcinogen (kar·SI·nuh·juhn): a substance that causes cancer.

cardiac output: the amount of blood pumped by your heart each minute.

cardiorespiratory (KAR·dee·oh·RES·puh·ruh·TOR·ee) **endurance:** the ability to stay active without getting tired.

career: the work that a person prepares for and does through life.

casual contact: daily contact without touching body fluids.

cat nap: a 20 to 30 minute nap during the day.

CD-ROM (SEE·DEE·RAHM): a computer disc that stores computer programs.

349

cell: the smallest living part of the body.

cerebellum (ser·uh·BEL·uhm): the part of the brain that controls how well your muscles work together.

cerebral palsy (suh·REE·bruhl PAHL·zee): a chronic disease that interferes with muscle coordination.

cerebrum (suh·REE·bruhm): the part of the brain that controls your ability to learn, your memory, and your voluntary muscle control.

certificate: a document issued by a nongovernment agency that states a person is qualified to perform a certain job.

character: the effort you use to act on responsible values.

choking: being unable to breathe.

chronic (KRAHN·ik) **health condition:** a condition that lasts a long time or keeps coming back.

cilia (SI·lee·uh): tiny hairs that line the air passages.

circulatory (SUHR·kyuh·luh·TOR·ee) **system:** the body system that transports oxygen, food, and waste through the body.

cirrhosis (suh·ROH·suhs): a disease in which liver cells are damaged.

clique (CLIK): a group of people who keep other people out of their group.

cocaine: an illegal stimulant made from coca bush leaves.

codeine (KOH·deen): a narcotic painkiller made from morphine.

cold: a respiratory infection caused by any of 200 different viruses.

commercial: an ad on television or radio.

communicable disease: a disease caused by pathogens that can be spread.

communication: an exchange of information with others.

complex carbohydrates: nutrients that provide long-lasting energy.

compliment: a positive statement about a person or his or her behavior.

compost (KAHM·post): dead plants and food that can be used to make living plants grow.

conflict: a disagreement.

conflict resolution skills: steps you can take to settle disagreements in a responsible way.

congenital (kuhn·JEN·uh·tuhl) **heart disease:** defects in the heart that are present at birth.

conservation: the saving of resources.

consumer: a person who judges information and buys products and services.

consumer complaint: a way of telling others that you are not happy with a product or service.

contact lenses: lenses that fit directly on the eye for clear vision.

cool-down: five to ten minutes of easy exercise after a workout.

coordination (KOH·OR·duh·NAY·shuhn): the ability to use body parts and senses together for movement.

couch potato: a person who is inactive.

crack: an illegal stimulant that is stronger than cocaine.

critical thinking skills: skills that help you think quickly and decide what to do.

cystic fibrosis (SIS·tik fy·BROH·sis): an inherited disease in which thick mucus clogs the lungs.

D

dandruff: flakes of dead skin cells on the scalp.

death: the loss of life when vital organs no longer work.

decibel (DE·suh·buhl): a measure of the loudness of sounds.

dental hygienist (DEN·tuhl hy·JE·nist): a person who works with a dentist to take care of patients' teeth.

deodorant (dee·OH·duh·ruhnt): a grooming product used under the arms to control body odor.

depressant: a drug that slows down body functions.

diabetes (DY·uh·BEE·teez): a disease in which the body does not make or cannot use insulin.

Dietary Guidelines: suggested goals for eating to help you stay healthy and live longer.

dietitian: a nutrition expert.

digestive system: the body system that breaks down food so that it can be used by the body.

discrimination: treating some people in a different way than you treat others.

distress: unsuccessful coping or a harmful response to a stressor.

divorce: a legal way to end a marriage.

drug: a substance that changes the way your body or mind works.

drug abuse: the use of an illegal drug or the harmful use of a legal drug on purpose.

drug addiction: a strong desire to take drugs even though drug use causes harm.

drug dependence: depending on drugs for their emotional or physical effects.

drug-free: to say NO to all harmful drug use.

drug misuse: the unsafe use of a legal drug that is not on purpose.

drug trafficking: the illegal purchase or sale of drugs.

E

earthquake: a violent shaking of Earth's surface.

eating disorder: a harmful way of eating because a person cannot cope.

emergency: a situation in which help is needed quickly.

emergency medical technician (tek·NI·shuhn) **(EMT):** a person who takes care of people in emergency situations before they reach the hospital.

emotions: the feelings you have inside you.

emphysema (EMP·fuh·ZEE·muh): a disease in which air sacs in the lungs are damaged.

endocrine (EN·duh·kruhn) **system:** the body system made up of glands.

energy: the ability to do work.

environment: everything that is around you.

Environmental Protection Agency (EPA): a government office that makes rules and enforces laws to help control pollution.

epilepsy (EP·uh·LEP·see): a chronic disease in which nerve messages in the brain are disturbed for brief periods of time.

ethnic food: a food eaten by people of a specific culture.

eustress (YOO·stres): a healthful response to a stressor.

expenses: products and services a person needs to buy.

F

fad: a style or product that is popular for a short time.

false claim: a statement that is not true.

family: the group of people to whom you are related.

family guideline: a rule set by your parents or guardian that helps you know how to act.

family value: the worth or importance of something to your family.

farsighted: having clear vision far away and blurred vision up close.

fast food restaurant: a place that serves food quickly.

Federal Trade Commission (FTC): a federal agency that deals with false advertising.

fetal (FEE·tuhl) **alcohol syndrome (FAS):** birth defects in babies whose mothers drank alcohol during pregnancy.

fever: a higher than normal body temperature.

fiber: the part of grains and plant foods that cannot be digested.

fighting: taking part in a physical struggle.

first aid: the temporary care given to a person who has a sudden illness or injury.

fitness skills: skills that can be used during physical activities.

FITT formula: a formula that tells you how to get fitness benefits from your workouts.

flexibility: the ability to bend and move your body easily.

flood: the overflowing of a body of water onto dry land.

flossing: a way to remove plaque and bits of food from between the teeth.

Food and Drug Administration (FDA): a federal agency that checks the safety and effectiveness of drugs and medical devices.

food group: foods that contain the same nutrients.

Food Guide Pyramid: a guide that shows how many servings are needed from each food group each day.

food label: a list of facts on a food container required by federal law.

foodborne illness: an illness caused by eating foods or drinking beverages that contain germs.

fossil fuels: coal, oil, and natural gas burned to make energy.

foster child: a child who lives in a family without being related by birth or adoption.

fracture: a break in a bone.

fungus (FUHN·guhs): a plant-like living thing.

G

gang: a group of people involved in dangerous and illegal actions.

gingivitis (jin·juh·VY·tuhs): a condition in which the gums are sore and bleed easily.

good character: telling the truth, showing respect, and being fair.

good sport: a person who respects others and follows safety rules for sports.

graffiti: markings on items that can be seen by others.

grains: seeds from certain plants.

gratitude: a feeling of thanks for a favor or for something that makes you happy.

grief (GREEF): discomfort that results from a loss.

grooming: taking care of your body and having a neat and clean appearance.

growth spurt (SPERT): a rapid increase in height and weight.

guidance counselor: a person who helps students solve problems, plan school subjects, and learn about careers.

Guidelines for Making Responsible Decisions™: questions you ask to help you make a responsible decision.

guilt: the bad feelings you get inside if you think or do something that you know is not right.

H

habit: a usual way of doing something.

hallucination: something that is seen or heard that is not real.

hallucinogens (huh·LOO·suhn·uh·juhnz): illegal drugs that cause hallucinations.

hashish (ha·SHEESH): a drug made from marijuana that has stronger effects.

hazardous waste: any substance that is harmful to people or animals.

health: the state of your body and mind and the way you get along with others.

health behavior contract: a written plan to practice a life skill.

health career: a job in the health field for which one trains.

health education teacher: a teacher who helps students develop health knowledge, practice life skills, and form healthful habits.

health fitness: having the heart, lungs, muscles, and joints in top condition.

health knowledge: an awareness of facts about health.

health product: an item that is used for physical, mental, or social health.

health service: a person or place that helps improve your physical, mental, or social health.

healthful behavior: an action that increases the level of health for you and others.

healthful TV programs: TV programs that promote physical, mental, or social health.

hearing aid: a device that makes sounds louder.

hearing loss: the inability to hear or interpret certain sounds.

heart attack: a sudden lack of oxygen to the heart.

heart disease: a disease of the heart and blood vessels.

heart rate: the number of times your heart beats each minute.

helper T cell: a white blood cell that helps make antibodies.

heredity: the traits that you get from your natural parents.

heroin (HEHR·uh·wuhn): an illegal narcotic made from morphine.

HIV: the pathogen that destroys helper T cells and causes AIDS.

honest talk: the open sharing of feelings.

hormone (HOR·mohn): a chemical that is produced by glands and controls body activities.

hurricane: a tropical storm with heavy rains and winds over 74 miles per hour.

I

I-message: a statement that includes a behavior, the effect of the behavior, and the feeling that results.

illegal drug use: using illegal drugs or using legal drugs in a way that breaks the law.

immune: to be protected from a certain disease.

incinerator (in·SI·nuh·RAY·ter): a furnace in which garbage and other wastes are burned.

income: the money a person receives or earns.

incubation (IN·kyuh·BAY·shuhn) **period:** the time from when a pathogen enters the body until symptoms of disease appear.

influenza (in·FLOO·en·suh) **(flu):** a viral infection of the respiratory tract.

ingredients (in·GREE·dee·uhnts) **listing:** the list of ingredients that are in the food or beverage.

inhalant (in·HAY·luhnt): a chemical that is breathed.

insulin: a hormone that helps body cells use sugar from foods.

involuntary muscles: muscles that work automatically.

isokinetic (eye·suh·ki·NE·tik) **exercise:** an exercise in which weight is moved through a full range of motion.

isometric (eye·suh·ME·trik) **exercise:** an exercise in which you contract your muscles without moving them.

isotonic (eye·suh·TAH·nik) **exercise:** an exercise in which you contract muscles to produce movement.

J-K-L

joint: a place where two bones meet.

justice: fairness for all people.

landfill: a place where waste is dumped and buried.

law: a rule that represents the beliefs of most people in a community, state, or nation.

learning disability: a disorder that causes someone to have difficulty learning.

learning style: the way you gain skills and information.

license: a document issued by a government agency that states a person can legally perform a certain job.

life cycle: the stages of life from birth to death.

life skill: a healthful action you learn and practice for the rest of your life.

lifestyle: your way of living.

ligaments (LIG·uh·muhnts): bands of tissue that hold bones together at movable joints.

litter: trash that is thrown on land or in water.

LSD: an illegal hallucinogen that causes flashbacks.

M

marijuana (MEHR·uh·WAH·nuh): an illegal drug that affects mood and short-term memory.

marriage: a legal commitment that a couple makes to love and care for one another.

mature: to become fully grown or developed.

media: ways of sending messages to consumers.

media literacy: being able to see and evaluate the messages you get from the media.

medical checkup: a series of tests that measure your health status.

medicine: a drug used to prevent, treat or cure a health condition.

medulla (muh·DUH·luh): the part of the brain that controls actions such as heart rate and breathing.

mental alertness: the sharpness of your mind.

mentor: a responsible person who helps a younger person.

mind-body connection: the idea that your thoughts and feelings have an effect on your body.

mood swings: changes in emotions caused by hormone levels.

morphine (MOR·feen): a narcotic used to control pain.

motivate: to encourage someone to do well.

mucus (MYOO·kuhs): a moist coating that lines your nose and throat.

muscle strain: an overstretch of a muscle.

muscular dystrophy (DIS·truh·fee): a disease in which muscles lose the ability to work.

muscular endurance: the ability to use the same muscles for a long period of time.

muscular strength: the amount of force your muscles can produce.

muscular system: the body system that helps you move and maintain posture.

mutual (MYOO·chuh·wuhl) **respect:** the high regard two people have for one another.

N

narcotic (nar·KAH·tik): a drug that slows down the nervous system and relieves pain.

nearsighted: having clear vision up close and blurred vision far away.

nervous system: the body system for communication and control.

nicotine (NI·kuh·TEEN): a stimulant drug found in tobacco.

noise pollution: loud or constant noise that causes hearing loss and stress.

nutrients: substances in food that your body uses for energy and for growth and repair of cells.

Nutrition Facts: a panel on a food label that gives facts about the food or beverage.

O

open dump: an area where garbage and wastes are piled.

ophthalmologist (ahf·thuh·MAHL·uh·jist): a physician who studies diseases and disorders of the eye.

opportunistic (AHP·uhr·too·NIST·ik) **disease:** a disease that would not occur if the body defenses were working normally.

optician (ahp·TI·shuhn): a person who grinds lenses and makes glasses.

optometrist (ahp·TAH·muh·trist): a person who is trained to examine eyes and diagnose and treat vision and eye problems.

organ: a group of tissues that work together.

orthodontist (or·thuh·DAHN·tist): a dentist who is trained to fit braces on people's teeth.

ovaries: the female reproductive glands that produce ova, or egg cells.

over-the-counter (OTC) drug: a medicine that you can buy without a doctor's order.

overfat: having too much body fat.

overweight: a weight above your healthful weight.

P

pancreas: a gland that produces insulin.

pathogen (PA·thuh·juhn): a germ that causes disease.

PCP: an illegal hallucinogen that speeds up and slows down the body.

peace: being without unsettled conflicts within yourself or with others.

pedestrian (puh·DES·tree·uhn): a person who walks on the sidewalk or in the street.

peer: a person who is about your age.

peer pressure: the influence that peers try to have on your decisions.

periodontal (per·ee·oh·DAHN·tuhl) **disease:** a disease of the gums and bone that support the teeth.

personal flotation device (PFD): a device that helps you stay afloat.

personal health record: written information about your health.

personality: a blend of the different traits you have.

perspiration (per·spuh·RAY·shuhn): a liquid produced in sweat glands.

physical fitness: having your body in top condition.

physician (fuh·ZI·shun): a medical doctor who is trained to diagnose and treat illnesses.

pituitary (puh·TOO·uh·TER·ee) **gland:** an endocrine gland that helps control growth rate.

plaque (PLAK): a sticky substance on teeth that contains bacteria.

poison: a substance that causes harm if it enters the body.

pollutant: something that has a harmful effect on the environment.

pollution (puh·LOO·shuhn): the presence of substances in the environment that can harm your health.

positive attitude: a positive way of thinking and seeing things.

positive environment: an environment that promotes physical, social, and mental health.

posture: the way you hold your body as you sit, stand, and move.

power: the ability to combine strength and speed.

precycling: taking actions to reduce waste.

premature death: a death that happens before the usual time.

premature heart disease: heart disease that occurs before old age.

prescription drug: a medicine that you can buy only if your doctor writes an order.

productive argument: a discussion of different viewpoints without fighting.

protozoa (PROH·tuh·ZOH·uh): tiny, single-celled animals.

psychologist (sy·KAH·luh·jist): a person who applies knowledge about the mind and ways people behave to help people solve problems.

puberty (PYOO·ber·tee): the stage in life when a person's body changes to be able to reproduce.

puncture (PUHNK·cher): a wound in which something goes deep through the skin and makes a hole.

Q

quackery (KWA·kuh·ree): a method of selling worthless products and services.

R

radon (RAY·dahn): a radioactive gas that you cannot see or smell.

reaction time: the length of time it takes to move after a signal.

recovery period: the time during which visible symptoms of disease go away but you are not back to full speed.

recovery program: a group that supports people who are trying to change.

recycling: changing waste products so they can be used again.

recycling center: a place where waste products are changed so they can be used again.

relationships: the connections you have with other people.

REM: the stage of sleep when you dream.

renewable energy: energy whose source can be replaced.

reputation: the quality of your character as judged by others.

resistance skills: skills that help you resist pressure to make a wrong decision.

respect: thinking highly of someone.

respiratory (RES·puh·ruh·TOR·ee) **system:** the body system that helps the body use the air you breathe.

responsible decision: a decision that is safe, healthful, and follows laws and family guidelines.

responsible value: a belief that guides you to behave in responsible ways.

rest: a period of relaxation.

resting heart rate: your heart rate when you are lying down or sitting quietly.

reusing: using items again instead of throwing them away and buying new ones.

rheumatic (roo·MAT·ik) **heart disease:** damage to the heart valves that occurs if strep throat is not treated.

RICE treatment: a treatment for injuries to muscles and bones.

rickettsia (ri·KET·see·uh): pathogens that grow inside living cells and resemble bacteria.

risk behavior: an action that can be harmful to you and others.

risk situation: a condition that can harm your health.

role model: a person whose behavior other people copy.

S

safety belt: the lap belt and the shoulder belt.

safety rules: guidelines to help prevent injury.

saturated (SA·chuh·RAYT·uhd) **fats:** fats in foods that come from animals.

school nurse: a nurse who works in a school and takes care of ill or injured students and teachers.

school psychologist (SY·KAH·luh·jist): a psychologist who is trained to work with students, teachers, and parents and guardians.

scoliosis (skoh·lee·OH·sis): a curving of the spine to one side of the body.

scrape: a wearing away of the outer layer of the skin.

sebaceous (si·BAY·shuhs) **glands:** oil glands that produce sebum.

sebum (SEE·buhm): an oily substance that keeps skin from drying.

secondhand smoke: exhaled smoke and sidestream smoke.

seizure (SEE·zhuhr): the period of time during which loss of control occurs.

self-control: the degree to which you regulate your behavior.

self-discipline: the effort you make to do something.

self-respect: the good feelings you have about yourself when you behave in responsible ways.

separation: a situation in which parents are married but living apart.

sewage: a waste material carried off by sewers.

sexually transmitted disease (STD): a disease caused by pathogens that are spread during sexual contact.

shadowing: spending time with a mentor as he or she performs work activities.

sidestream smoke: smoke from a burning cigarette or cigar.

sign language: a way of communicating in which the fingers and hands are used instead of the spoken word.

skeletal system: the body system that forms a framework to support the body and to help protect internal soft tissues.

sleep: deep relaxation in which you are not aware of what is happening around you.

sleep cycle: the stages your body goes through while you sleep.

smoke detector: a device that sends a signal when smoke is present.

smokeless tobacco: tobacco that is chewed.

social skills: skills that help you interact with others.

sore throat: a sore or scratchy throat.

speed: the ability to move quickly.

spinal cord: a thick band of nerve cells through which messages enter and leave the brain.

sports checkup: a series of tests you have before you can play sports.

sprain: an injury to the tissue that connects bones to a joint.

steroids (STEHR·oydz)**:** drugs that act like hormones.

stimulant (STIM·yuh·luhnt)**:** a drug that speeds up the body functions.

stomach acids: kill pathogens that are swallowed.

strep throat: a bacterial infection of the throat.

stress: the body's reaction to the demands of daily living.

stress management skills: ways to reduce harmful effects of body changes caused by a stressor.

stressor: something that causes stress.

support network: the group of people who care about you.

symptom: a change in your behavior or a body function.

T

table manners: polite ways to eat.

tamper-resistant seal: an unbroken seal to show a container has not been opened.

target heart rate: a fast and safe heart rate for workouts to get cardiorespiratory endurance.

tears: coat your eyes each time you blink.

tendons (TEN·duhnz)**:** tough tissue fibers that connect muscles to bones.

testes (TES·teez)**:** the male reproductive glands that produce sperm cells.

tetanus (TET·nuhs)**:** an infection caused by poisons from bacteria that have entered the body.

time management plan: a plan that shows how a person will spend time.

tissue: a group of cells that work together.

tobacco: a plant that contains nicotine.

tobacco cessation (se·SAY·shuhn) **program:** a program to quit tobacco use.

tobacco-free: to say NO to using tobacco and to breathing smoke from tobacco products.

tolerance: a condition in which more of a drug is needed to get the same effects.

tornado: a violent, spinning wind-storm that has a funnel-shaped cloud.

toxic waste: waste that is poisonous.

tranquilizer (TRAN·kwuh·LY·zuhr): a drug that relieves anxiety.

tutor: a person who gives individual help to a student.

U

unbroken skin: blocks pathogens from entering your body.

unconscious (uhn·KAHN·shuhs): the condition of not being aware of surroundings.

undercurrent: a strong current under the surface of the water.

underweight: a weight below your healthful weight.

unique (yoo·NEEK): one of a kind.

universal precautions: steps taken to keep from having contact with pathogens in body fluids.

unsafe touch: a touch that is not right.

unsaturated fats: fats in foods that come from vegetables, nuts, seeds, poultry, and fish.

V

vaccine (vak·SEEN): a medicine that has dead or weak pathogens in it.

vein: a blood vessel that carries blood to the heart.

ventricles (VEN·tri·kuhlz): the lower parts of the heart.

victim of violence: a person who is harmed by violence.

violence: an act that harms oneself, others, or property.

virus (VY·ruhs): a pathogen that makes copies of itself.

visual environment: everything a person sees regularly.

visual pollution: sights that are unattractive.

voluntary muscles: muscles that you control.

volunteer: a person who provides a service without being paid.

W-X-Y-Z

wanna-be: a young person who is not yet a gang member but wants to be one.

warm-up: three to five minutes of easy physical activity before a workout.

water-treatment plant: a place where water from nearby rivers and streams is made safe to drink.

weapon: a device used for violence.

Web site: a collection of files or "pages" kept on a computer.

weight management: a plan used to have a healthful weight.

wellness: the highest level of health you can reach.

white blood cell: a blood cell that helps destroy pathogens.

withdrawal symptoms: unpleasant reactions when a drug is no longer taken.

World Wide Web (Web): a computer system that lets you find information, pictures, and text.

wrong decision: a decision that is harmful, unsafe, and breaks laws or family guidelines.

Gingivitis, 142

Glands

  pituitary, 80

  sebaceous, 144

Good character, 18

Good sport, 159

Grains, 105; 107

Gratitude, 19

Grief, 90

Grooming, 144

Growth spurt, 86

Guidance counselor, 274

Guidelines for Making Responsible Decisions™, 13

Guilt, 64

Guns, 332

H

Habit, 58

Hair care, 144

Hallucinogens, 209

Handwashing, 220

Hashish, 207

Hazardous waste, 285

Health, 5

Health behavior contract, 10

Health career, 270

Health careers, 270–275

Health education teacher, 273

Health fitness, 148

Health information, 256–257

Health knowledge, 6

Health product, 252

Health service, 253

Healthful behavior, 5

Hearing aid, 138

Hearing loss, 138; 289

Heart, and exercise, 152; 231

Heart attack, 230

Heart disease, 229–231

Heart murmur, 229

Heart rate, 152; 160

Helper T cell, 243

Hepatitis A, 219

Hepatitis B, 218

Heredity, 58; 126

Heroin, 205

High blood pressure, 230

"High on Health," 4–11

HIV, 65; 242–247; 336

Honest talk, 41; 183

Hormone, 80

Hurricane, 317

I

Illegal drug use, 202–209

I-message, 27